THE MAGIC OF BAKING SODA

By Emily Thacker

Published by:

James Direct Inc

500 S. Prospect Ave.

Hartville, Ohio 44632

U.S.A.

This book is intended as a record of folklore and historical solutions and is composed of tips, suggestions, and remembrances. It is sold with the understanding that the publisher is not engaged in rendering medical advice and does not intend this as a substitute for medical care by qualified professionals. No claims are intended as to the safety, or endorsing the effectiveness, of any of the remedies which have been included and the publisher cannot guarantee the accuracy or usefulness of individual remedies in this collection.

If you have a medical problem you should consult a physician.

Not For Resale

ISBN: 978-1-62397-037-6

Printing 12 11 10 9 8 7 6

First Edition   **Copyright 2010**   **James Direct Inc**

Table of Contents

Dear Reader,

It is a joy to come to you again with another collection of old-time home remedies.

I cannot begin to tell you how many kind readers have written to me, asking when the sequel to *THE VINEGAR HOME GUIDE* would appear. Your letters have been a real encouragement! Many of you have also shared your remembrances, and commented on the cleaning tips you found to be most useful.

One theme keeps reoccurring in your letters. Readers, from all across the country, relate how baking soda is a part of better health and easier cleaning. As I read your letters I see a continuing concern for maintaining good health without a lot of prescription drugs and doctor visits. This book offers me the opportunity to share some ways that baking soda is used to aid health and well being.

My mail also shows you have many unanswered questions about how baking soda cleans, how it can be used around the home and what part it plays in maintaining a healthy body. As always, my first consideration in bringing cleaning tips and remedies to you is:

Could this do harm?

Is it safe?

Is it time tested?

Beyond that, much of what this book does is relate the history of how people across the world, and down through time, have found baking soda to be useful in their daily lives.

4

Over the years, my fascination with all things natural and kind to the body and environment encouraged me to gather this collection of cleaning, cooking and health lore. Many of these hints and tips work wonders – in a particular situation. In other circumstances they may be less effective. A lot depends on the specific cleaning chore or body concern. I invite you to enjoy reading the cleaning tips and healing remedies in this book to see how others have used baking soda.

Then, I encourage you to experiment to find what works best for you. You may find the most helpful tip to be the way baking soda helps to clean and deodorize pets, the way baking soda can lead you to better health, how it cleans around the home or you may find you like the special, zesty taste it brings to baked goods. Whatever the reason you find for appreciating the many benefits of baking soda, I think you will find it a great companion book to the others in my series of books on natural healing and old-time ways of healing.

Like all old-time wisdom that is handed down from one generation to the next, many uses are very helpful today. Still, others may not be the best solution in today's world. Be sure to talk to your healthcare practitioner before making regular use of any home remedy, whether it is baking soda, vinegar or any other food or substance.

You asked for it! A special thank you to the many readers who have shared home remedies and cleaning tips they and their families use. You have shown me that baking soda has uncountable uses in and around the home, as well as in and outside the body. Because of its amazing healing properties over hundreds of years, it has sometimes been called the family's drugstore in a handy box!

I believe it was the German poet Goethe who wrote, "If everyone would sweep the street in front of their own house, the whole world would be clean." To paraphrase that philosophy, I believe that if we each protect our own little corner of the earth, the entire planet will be safe. To this end, most of the cleaning tips in this volume recommend using scraps of old cloth for cleaning rather than paper towels. Paper cleaning products are handy things, and wonderful for really nasty cleanups.

But please remember, every time you use a paper towel, somewhere, a tree is cut down. Besides, cloth is reusable and so is less expensive, as well as being softer and less likely to scratch fine finishes.

Please remember, this book is an attempt to share information. The use of baking soda to clean will not disturb the environment, set off allergic reactions, pollute the air we breathe or deliver harsh chemicals to skin and air. But, even this remarkable substance has its limitations. Use it wisely. And, consider this volume as your open sesame to ... The incredible, edible, wonder of baking soda!

Wishing you all the best,

Emily Thacker

Emily Thacker

INTRODUCTION

Baking soda is a wonderfully safe, totally organic product that is a naturally occurring mineral. It is so safe you could eat an entire teaspoon of it, and it would not poison you.

That familiar yellow box of baking soda is an inexpensive, even cheap, product that is kind to the environment. Chemically, it reacts as if it were an alkali and is called bicarbonate of soda or sodium bicarbonate. Baking soda is also known as bicarbonate of soda, sodium bicarbonate, bread soda, sodium hydrogen carbonate or sodium acid carbonate.

Plain sodium carbonate is the product we know as washing soda. Washing soda is about four times as strong as baking soda. They are both processed from soda ash. It has a long history of usefulness and is most commonly seen as a white, crystalline powder.

Baking soda has a slight alkaline taste. It cleans and deodorizes your home, soothes both the inside and outside of your body, cares for your pets and helps in the yard and garden and activates some home water softeners.

Baking soda is a chemical compound, meaning it is made up of chemical elements that can be separated into simpler substances by chemical reactions. The naturally forming crystals of baking soda are ground into the fine powder we use for baking and cleaning.

Today, almost all baking soda is mined from trona ore, much of it from a huge deposit in the state of Wyoming. This one, 24 square mile mine, produces most of the world's soda.

Soda helps in making soap and detergents and is used in the process of refining aluminum and other metals. It is an important part of tanning leather, oil well drilling, rubber and plastic manufacturing, paper making and processing of textiles. Glass, such as that in home windows across the world, is produced when soda ash and sand are first heated, then quickly cooled. This method produces glass that is both durable and quite clear.

Baking soda has proved to be useful in neutralizing the effect of the white phosphorus that is used in incendiary bullets. Its use helps to prevent that horribly corrosive chemical from spreading inside a wound.

Baking soda is also used to treat the metabolic acidosis caused by renal failure. It is also used to treat aspirin and tricyclic antidepressant overdoses. These treatments are only used in a tightly controlled hospital situations.

Sodium bicarbonate is an acid salt that reacts with other chemicals as a mild alkali. It is extracted from soda ash, one form of which is the fine white powder that forms when wood or coal is burned. For commercial production sulfuric acid, coal and limestone can be combined to produce a reliable amount of soda ash. Another method that has been used to produce soda ash combines carbonic acid and sodium hydroxide. Read more about the production of baking soda later, in Chapter One.

Baking Soda As Leavening
If you were to put a small mound of baking soda in the oven, on a tray, and begin heating it, at about 150°F it would begin to become unstable and a little carbon

dioxide might slowly begin to seep out. As the heat increased, the compound would become more unstable and by the time it reached 300°F most of its available carbon dioxide would have been released.

For most of us, the first use of baking soda that comes to mind is as a leavening agent in baked goods. Because of the fact that when plain, dry baking soda is heated above 300°F, it releases carbon dioxide gas. This property is at the heart of many cooking uses of baking soda.

This means that any baked food that depends on baking soda for its leavening must be cooked at more than 300°F or the carbon dioxide releasing action does not fully take place. To allow for differences in ovens, most baking soda leavened cakes, biscuits and cookies are baked at a minimum of 350°F.

Baking soda will also release carbon dioxide in another way. If it comes into contact with an acid containing liquid, they immediately react. You can see this reaction by dropping a few drops of lemon juice or vinegar onto a teaspoon of baking soda.

Both of these ways of getting soda to release carbon dioxide gas serve to put bubbles of air into a batter or dough. Because of the way baking soda releases its leavening gas, soda containing products need to be cooked immediately after mixing to maximize the results of the carbon dioxide gas produced. If permitted to set for a lengthy time before baking the gas dissipates and the baked product will not rise properly.

Baking soda and its baking soda containing cousin, baking powder, are the basis for what are called quick breads because they do not rely on the time consuming process of rising that yeast based foods do. Baking soda leavens two ways:

- When combined with something acidic, carbon dioxide is released.

- When heated, carbon dioxide is released.

More About Baking Soda

How intensely acid a compound is, or how intensely based a compound may be is measured using the pH scale. The scale runs from 1 to 14, with 1 indicating a strong acid and 14 indicating a strong base (alkali). Distilled water, with a pH of 7, is considered neutral. Baking soda has a pH of 8.1, so it is a mild base. It tends to maintain its ph of 8.1, even if a small amount of an acid or base is added to it. This makes it ideal for controlling environments where ph stability is important. Soda's use in maintaining desired pH in swimming pools is a perfect example of this use.

In tooth paste and mouthwash products baking soda serves as an anti plaque agent. A good brightening and plaque fighting tooth paste can be made at home by combining hydrogen peroxide, baking soda and ..

Because of baking soda's crystalline structure, when used dry or as a paste, it is a gentle abrasive that removes dirt without leaving scratches in surfaces. Combine it with salt for a slightly more aggressive cleaner.

Coffee makers often get a build up of minerals in their water heating chamber. Running a strong baking soda solution through them can help to remove them and extend the life of the machine. It will also keep mineral build up from affecting the taste of the coffee. This is also a good treatment for espresso machines.

Baking soda works to neutralize odors by combining chemically with them, rather than simply masking them or absorbing them. This property is one of the reasons that a mixture of baking soda, hydrogen peroxide and hand soap makes a good mixture for removing skunk odor from pets' fur.

Because the carbon dioxide that baking soda releases when heated is heavier than air, it smothers fire. It covers the fire with a layer of gas that does not permit it access to the oxygen it needs to continue burning. Although it is useful on small grease fires, it should not be tossed on a deep fryer or any large container of oil. When baking soda is thrown on oil it will cause it to spatter and so spread the fire, as well as pose a danger to anyone close enough to do the tossing.

Controlling air pollution is made easier and less expensive with the use of baking soda because it has the ability to absorb sulfur dioxide, as well as other dangerous gases. It is also useful in pulling lead and other heavy metals from drinking water.

Medically Speaking
Baking soda has been used for hundreds of years to soothe the misery of itchy skin and the pain of insect bites. And, our ancestors were quite familiar with its ability to relieve the discomfort of too much acid in the stomach. Now, our more high tech medical world is using it to complement the latest medical treatments.

The prestigious *Journal of the American Society of Nephrology* reports that patients with chronic kidney disease can slow the progression of their renal failure by taking daily supplements of baking soda. This, doctors have found, works because a common complication of chronic kidney disease is a condition called metabolic

11

acidosis. This shortage of plasma bicarbonate can be relieved by taking baking soda on a daily basis.

Surprisingly, these kidney disease patients found that the baking soda supplements did not cause increased blood pressure from the increased sodium intake. Nor did these patients suffer from an increase in ankle or leg swelling from the extra sodium in their diets.

Researchers also found that overall nutrition values improved in these patients. Their improved overall health led to a dramatic lessening of their likelihood of requiring dialysis.

Another way baking soda is used by the medical profession that impacts the kidneys is as a carrier for the contrast dye that is injected before CT scans or X rays.

Previously, a saline solution was used to carry the dye, by IV line, into the body. New research shows that a baking soda solution is much safer for the health of the kidneys. The saline (salt) based solution has been shown to sometimes cause the kidneys to allow protein normally kept in the blood plasma to leak into the urine. This drop in blood protein leads to fluid leaking from the blood stream, resulting in tissue swelling.

Baking soda baths are high on the list of comfort strategies doctors recommend for patients with primary biliary cirrhosis. As the cirrhosis advances, itching can become a major symptom. Generous amounts of baking soda, added to a cool bath, is one of the first methods doctors suggest for relieving this intense itching. They also recommend following standard shampooing with a rinse of baking soda and water.

Baking Soda In The Laundry Room

Soda is often added to laundry detergents to prevent the minerals in hard water from bonding with the actual detergent, making it less effective. Soda also helps to remove alcohol and grease stains from clothing.

When about a third of a cup of baking soda is added to a washer load of clothes the amount of bleach needed to remove stains is cut in half.

Baking soda's mild alkalinity turns fatty acids, such as grease, into soap that can then be dissolved in water and rinsed away.

If you want to save big dollars in the laundry room you might want to entirely eliminate buying laundry detergent. Instead, try this:

1   Teaspoon grated hand soap
1   Teaspoon baking soda
2   Teaspoons borax

Just add this mixture to a hot water wash and clothes will be clean, fresh smelling and odor free. If you are concerned that this seems to be a much smaller amount of cleaning product than you usually add to your laundry, remember that both liquid and powdered detergents contain large amounts of inert fillers. For example, consider how much actual detergent you would be adding to your wash if all the water was removed from your favorite liquid detergent! Measured by weight, the amount of fillers in dry detergents varies from brand to brand, but can go as high 85% of the total weight.

HHO Fuel

HHO fuel gets its name from H-2-0, which means plain old water. Both baking soda and its stronger cousin washing soda have been lauded as useful ingredients in schemes to permit cars to run on water rather than gasoline or diesel fuel. These fuel conversion proposals are usually based on the theory that says electricity from a car's battery can be used to convert water into hydrogen and oxygen gases. Then, they propose, it is possible to burn these two gases as a supplement to ordinary fuel.

It sounds like a reasonable theory. In practice, it is not so reasonable. The entire retro fitting of a car to produce and utilize this system can cost $2,000 or more. The amount of gases actually produced is too tiny to, in the real world, affect mileage. It looks like you might want to save that new box of baking soda for scrubbing away greasy dirt on your hubcaps!

Buying Baking Soda

Be sure to be a comparison shopper when buying baking soda. Compare prices for baking soda, even within the same store. Sometimes the big box of baking soda in the soap and detergent aisle actually costs more per ounce than the small box of baking soda you find in the baking products aisle! And, soda for baking is more likely to be available as a low cost generic than the same baking soda aimed at the laundry market. Therefore, buy with care.

And now, as you read the rest of this book, may you find that baking soda is definitely an ...

... Incredible, Edible, Wonder!

Chapter One

THE FASCINATING HISTORY OF BAKING SODA!

Throughout the ancient world, hot springs were valued for their healing powers. Many of these springs contain fairly high concentrations of sodium bicarbonate. These soda laden waters, wherever they were found in the world, drew people suffering from a wide array of physical and mental complaints. Some of the most famous include those in:

- Afyon, Turkey, where the water is said to be helpful for those suffering from arthritis, sciatica, back pain, muscle and nerve fatigue, neuritis, neuralgia or lumbago. The baths there are also locally recommended for anyone who has had recent surgery of any kind. It has also been said to provide relief for those with psoriasis, eating problems, stomach, intestine, gall bladder, kidney, urinary tract and gynecologic disorders.

- Hot Springs, Arkansas, where the waters have drawn thousands of visitors who believe in their healing effects. They are said to be useful for those with muscle problems, cardiovascular disease and nervous system imbalances.

- Inyo/Tecopa Springs, California, located in

the Mojave Desert, where research on the whole-body benefits of hot springs is being studied.

- Jiaosi Hot Springs in Taiwan, where their particularly clear springs are clear and odorless and promise to leave the visitor with especially smooth skin. The soda fortified water here is considered to be able to revitalize the entire body when one drinks the water.

- Spain is famous for bicarbonate springs that are used to open peripheral blood vessels to improve circulation to the body's extremities.

- Other European springs are believed to be helpful to those with hypertension and atherosclerosis.

History of Baking Soda

Many hot mineral springs contain lots of sodium bicarbonate. Sometimes it crystallizes around the edges, making naturally occurring hot springs a valuable source of soda for many of the world's oldest cultures. These springs, with their high mineral content, were the perfect environment for soda to effervesce, or evaporate out, and settle in crystals around the outside borders. Almost everywhere hot springs with high sodium bicarbonate levels occur there is a history of people collecting it by scraping up the loose crystals as they formed on the outside ring of the water pools.

Soda And Soap

Ever wonder what that familiar arm and hammer on the box of a popular brand of baking soda stands for? It is intended to represent Vulcan, the Roman god of the forge and of fire. Perhaps that was chosen because another early source of soda ash, or the white powder formed when wood is thoroughly burned, was from the residue of cooking and heating fires.

Inscriptions on urns that date back to about 2800 BC tell of their use for holding a mixture of ashes and animal fat. This nearly 50 centuries old production method may have resulted in a very crude soap, but it was a beginning.

Folklore says that using sodium carbonate and sodium bicarbonate to make soap was revealed to mankind after burnt offerings were made to various deities. The learning process began when women who were washing clothes in a river discovered that one particular area of water got their laundry cleaner and sometimes would even produce a foamy substance.

What happened was that above that area of the river animal sacrifices were burnt. The fat from the sacrifices would drip into the hot ashes, forming soap. Add in a little rain and the crude soap would seep down the hill, over the riverbank and into the water. Eventually someone figured out what was happening and then everyone could make soap whenever they wanted to.

Folklore may not have gotten it exactly right, but soap making WAS developed many centuries ago. Today, many different kinds of oils are used to replace the animal fat that was once cooked to extract its oil:

- Olive oil produces a very mild soap.

- Coconut oil produces lots of foam.

- Palm oil is used to make soap hard.

Today's best soaps often contain a mixture of these ingredients, along with a wide variety of flower and herb scents.

Mining and Manufacturing Soda

The soda ash the makes baking soda can come into being in several ways. It is the soft white powder that forms when wood or coal is burned. It can even be formed by burning plants or processing table salt. An ancient method of obtaining soda ash was to burn seaweed.

Leblanc process for soda ash This outdated method of producing soda ash was one of the first commercial ways of obtaining large amounts of it. Salt (sodium chloride) was heated with sulfuric acid. This dangerous combination produced sodium sulfate and hydrochloric acid. Once the sulfuric acid was pulled out the sodium sulfate was heated with coal and limestone to produce the soda ash.

Solvay process for soda ash Because of the corrosive acids associated with the Leblanc process, a less dangerous process was needed for producing soda ash. This newer process also begins with plain old table salt. The salt is turned into a concentrated slurry, then carbon dioxide and ammonia are run through it. This causes crude sodium bicarbonate to precipitate out when it is heated.

Both of these old processes resulted in dangerous by-products that had serious disposal problems. Eventually, trona ore, which is nearly pure sodium carbonate, was discovered.

Small beds of trona ore, or soda ash, have been identified in many countries across the world. These places include such diverse areas as Botswana, Turkey, Egypt, Kenya and Namibia. These are all small deposits and are nowhere near able to supply the world's need for soda, which is why the complicated Leblanc and Solvay processes were needed.

Then, in the 1930s, the entire idea of soda production changed. A huge deposit of very pure trona ore was discovered in Wyoming. Called the Green River Formation, this nearly pure soda deposit covers more than 24 square miles. It is the residue of what was once thought to be a 600 square mile body of water that, over the eons, evaporated and left behind 200 billion tons of trona ore.

Huge sheets of ore are layered between bands of sandstone and shale. It is estimated that this one deposit will be able to supply the world's soda ash needs for thousands of years.

The gigantic mine that is the Green River Formation is more than 1,500 feet deep and contains 2,500 miles of tunnels. It covers two dozen square miles with its maze of 15 foot wide, 9 foot tall tunnels.

Processing Trona Ore
Basically, trona ore is processed simply by dissolving it in water and bubbling carbon dioxide through it. Steps to turn the ore into food grade baking soda:

- Mix the ore with water to form a slurry (at this point it is technically called sodium sesquicaronate).

- Spin the liquid in a centrifuge to form a combination of liquid and crystals.

- Dissolve the crystals in a rotating dissolver to form a saturated solution that is filtered to remove all non soluble impurities.

- Carbon dioxide is introduced and soda crystals precipitate out of the solution, ready to be dried and ground into powder.

This process does not produce the large amounts of toxic by-products of other methods and results in an extremely pure product.

Chapter Two

AROUND THE HOME

Sodium bicarbonate, or baking soda, has been around since the beginning of time! It is a naturally occurring mineral that is both safe on the environment as well as inexpensive to purchase. With its seemingly endless list of uses, baking soda is as economical as it is versatile! From being used as a leavening agent to helping delicious baked goods rise to its use as an antacid ... and even its use in cleaning the Statue of Liberty ... baking soda's uses seem endless. But baking soda is also one of the most versatile cleaning agents around!!!

DID YOU KNOW?

- Baking soda tends not to dissolve in alcohol.

- Alka Seltzer® is baking soda combined with citric acid.

- Large particles of baking soda were used to clean the Statue of Liberty.

- Contrary to urban legend, baking soda and bleach do not explode. They actually enhance each other's actions.

WHY BAKING SODA?

Unlike most commercial household chemicals

and cleaners, baking soda is a mineral found abundantly in nature that is in just about every living thing. It is a safe, natural substance that has been used for centuries in everything from cleaning to bathing to cooking. Baking soda is safe enough to eat. How many of your household cleaners or commercial chemicals can claim the same thing?

Baking soda can be found in all your favorite recipes for baked goods like muffins, cakes and cookies!!

Baking soda can be used to brush your teeth...

You can bathe in baking soda...

NO household commercial cleaners can boast such a statement! In fact, just the opposite! Many household cleaners we use every day can actually be harmful to both body and environment!

Dangerous Toxins

Many of the store bought cleaning agents that we have come to depend on to clean our homes are made from chemicals that could actually be harmful to our health! Dangerous chemicals can be found in the very products we are purchasing to clean our homes. Cleaners are filled with ingredient after ingredient of chemical compounds and derivatives that we cannot even pronounce. Yet we squirt them on our counters, spray them on our mirrors, rinse them through our clothing and wipe them onto our cups and dishes!

These chemicals are being used on a daily basis in the confines of our homes without the benefit of fresh air circulation to help dilute their potentially toxic effects. And, science is still studying the effects of long term exposure on our bodies to these household chemicals. A few of the questions being asked about household cleaners and commercial chemicals include:

- What are the long term health risks to my body from chemical exposure?

- Will germs become resistant to chemicals found in my cleaner?

- What happens if I mix dangerous cleaning chemicals together?

- What if my child or grandchild gets into my household cleaning products?

- Is there a link between the chemicals found in every day cleaning products and cancer, birth defects or fertility problems?

- Do store bought cleaning agents cause asthma or allergies?

Chemical Cleaners and the Environment

Consumers are also becoming more aware of the potential impact commercial chemical cleaners have on our environment. Many consider household cleaners to be detrimental to the environment. Consider:

- Pollution is created in the manufacturing of both chemical-based cleaning products and the plastic bottles themselves.

- Millions of plastic bottles and containers wind up in landfills.

- Many of the chemical compounds in household cleaners have been found to harm wildlife as they are eventually added to our waste systems.

- Chemical elements from discarded cleaners and runoff waste have shown up in our streams and wetlands affecting the fish and game population.

Cost of Store Bought Cleaning Agents
The household cleaning industry is a 14+ billion dollar a year business! Each year, the cleaning industry offers dozens of "new and improved" products we MUST have, if our homes are to be "genuinely" clean and disinfected. How much money do we spend on everyday household cleaners?

Billions of advertising dollars are spent by corporations to get you to buy a commercial cleaner from them, while we already have our very own, natural cleaning solutions right in our own kitchen pantry! And our old-school cleaners are natural, proven safe to use and cost only pennies!

Today, more and more of us are opting out of purchasing high-cost chemical cleaners with unknown potential health risks and choosing a natural cleaning alternative in the power of baking soda! It is natural and costs almost nothing to use! Think of all the separate cleaners we purchase to clean particular areas of our home:

- Kitchen cleaners

- Bathroom floors

- Tub and tile

- Carpet and rug deodorizers

- Appliance polish

24

- Drain cleaners

- Laundry detergent

- Spot and stain removers

- Toilet bowl cleaner

- Air fresheners

- Scouring powders

- Degreasers

- Window and mirror cleaners

- Furniture polish

And, the list goes on!

Instead of purchasing a separate cleaner made for each different cleaning application, baking soda can be used to clean every area of your home! And, unlike mixing some store bought chemicals with bleach, you don't need to worry about dangerous fumes when combining baking soda and bleach for cleaning. In fact, baking soda and bleach combined actually enhance each other's cleaning action!

Next time you pick up that rag to clean, try a few of these cleaning solutions!

KITCHENS, BATHROOMS AND LIVING AREAS

Kitchens, bathrooms and other living rooms are high traffic areas for germs and dirt. These are the areas where we spend the majority of our time. They are where our children play and sleep. Instead of reaching for the latest, new and improved commercial cleaner, try natural baking soda! It will not leave a long-lasting chemical residue on the areas you live in most!

Small Appliances

Rub baking soda on the outside of your deep fryer to loosen grease and oil deposits; also good for cleaning electric can openers and toasters.

Baking soda is a good copper cleaner. It was even used on the inside copper walls of the Statue of Liberty!

Clean greasy appliances by wiping them down with a mixture of baking soda and vinegar.

Coffee Pots

Clean stained coffee pots with a solution of baking soda and warm water. For extra tough stains, let the coffee pot soak for at least an hour or two in between scrubs.

For periodic cleaning, add a few tablespoons of baking soda to your coffee maker and run it through the normal cycle.

Mineral deposits can be rinsed clean from your coffee maker by filling it with 1 cup of vinegar and 1/8 cup of baking soda. Boil the solution in the pot and allow it all to stand for about 10 minutes. Be sure to rinse the pot well.

Microwaves

Use baking soda sprinkled on a damp sponge to clean and remove food spills on the inside of a microwave.

Oven Cleaner

Sprinkle a 1/4 inch covering of baking soda over a

dirty oven and spray it with water. Let set until dry and re-spray. When dry, scoop the soda out and it will have soaked up spilled grease and baked on food deposits.

Exhaust Hoods

Clean kitchen stove exhaust hoods by adding a generous amount of soda to your cleaning water to cut the grease; helps cut through grease when cleaning kitchen walls, too.

Dishwashers

Clean your dishwasher by running through the wash and rinse cycles with baking soda spread in the unit. This will both clean and freshen your dishwasher.

Refrigerators and Freezers

Refrigerator and freezer door gaskets will last longer if cleaned only with a baking soda and water solution. Harsh cleaners and bleach can shorten their life.

The outside doors of your refrigerator or oven can be kept clean with a mixture of baking soda and water. Simply add to a damp sponge or cloth and wipe clean!

Deep clean your refrigerator of lingering smells and odors. Use baking soda as a cleansing powder by sprinkling it on a clean, damp sponge. Wipe down the inside of the refrigerator, being sure to reach all areas including shelves and bins. Include a fresh, opened box of soda to help absorb future odors when you are finished!

Strong, pungent refrigerator odors such as fish or sour milk can be eliminated by wiping any spills with a dampened sponge sprinkled with baking soda and vinegar. Absorb any lingering odors by placing an uncovered dish of fresh baking soda in the affected area.

Ranges

Ceramic cook tops on ranges can become caked with burned food dripped from pots and pans. Clean like new again by making a paste from baking soda and a small amount of water. Rub burned area with this mild abrasive until clean.

Cooked-on grease and food stains on your range or stovetop can be easily removed. Wet stained area with a damp sponge. Add a layer of baking soda and rub in a circular motion until clean.

Sinks and Countertops

Use baking soda in the place of powdered cleansers to clean porcelain or stainless steel kitchen and bathroom fixtures.

Add baking soda to your water for an all-over fresh cleaning for kitchens and bathrooms.

Use baking soda to clean kitchen countertops after cooking to clean and disinfect.

Marble countertops can be buffed new again by lightly dusting with baking soda and wiping with a damp, soft cloth. Let film dry for about 20 minutes before cleaning with a wet rag.

For difficult countertop stains, add a few drops of bleach to a baking soda paste. Rub paste with bleach into stain in a circular motion. Rinse area clean and dry.

Scrub stainless steel sinks with baking soda to make them shine without the danger of scratching them with a more abrasive substance. Baking soda is also good for cleaning stainless faucets, sink, stove, dish washer, microwave, toaster and refrigerator trims.

Wipe off the inside of kitchen cupboards with a damp towel and baking soda.

Remove knife scratches from countertops with a mixture of 1/4 cup baking soda and 6 or 7 tablespoons of water. Rub it into small scratches to smooth out surfaces.

Cutting Boards and Butcher's Blocks
Wipe down your kitchen cutting board with baking soda to neutralize odors after chopping onions, garlic, chives or other foods with strong flavors.

Periodically clean your plastic cutting board by scrubbing it with a combination of baking soda, salt and a little hot water.

After cutting fish, chicken or any meat, cover your kitchen cutting board with soda and let set for a few minutes. Rinse with vinegar to complete the disinfecting process.

Wooden butcher blocks and knife blocks can be disinfected and deodorized by washing them down with a mixture of baking soda and vinegar. Sprinkle baking soda on a vinegar soaked sponge or cloth and rub clean.

Dishes and Silverware
Scour out stained cups with baking soda...and don't forget the teapot, too.

Clean stained ceramic glasses and cups with a bit of baking soda on a damp cloth. This procedure is safe for your best china.

Lots of dirty dishes to wash? Add a handful of soda to the water and your detergent will work better and last longer!

Use baking soda to clean silver, with no hard rubbing or polishing.

Baking soda and water can be used as a soak and cleaner for silver. The soda works well, but beware of possible fumes!

Add a quarter cup of baking soda to dish water to get dishes really clean and sparkling.

Try baking soda on extra greasy dishes or pots and pans.

Add a couple of tablespoons of baking soda to your dishwasher for brighter, cleaner glassware and dishes.

Pots and Pans

Pots and pans that are really dirty can be cleaned like new with a solution of baking soda, vinegar and hot water. Let the pans soak in the solution for ten minutes before scrubbing clean.

Re-season Teflon®, Silverstone® and other non-stick surfaces by putting a cup of water in the pan and bringing to a boil. Add a couple of tablespoons of baking soda and a half cup of white vinegar and simmer for 8 – 12 minutes. Rinse the pan, dry it and wipe it down with olive oil.

Removing stains from non-stick cookware can be difficult without damaging the finish. For a safe way to get off tough stains safely, use a cup of boiling water with 3 tablespoons of baking soda and 1/2 cup of vinegar. Boil for 5 minutes, and then wash. After drying with a soft towel, wipe it down with vegetable or olive oil.

Baking soda and water can clean cast iron pots so that they look new again.

For tough stains on cast iron pots, boil 2 cups of water and 2 tablespoons of baking soda for 5 – 6 minutes. Empty and sprinkle baking soda into the wet pot. Scrub clean with plastic netting or a coarse sponge. Rinse out and wipe dry. Add a few drops of peanut oil to bring back the finish and to re-season the pan.

For a pan with baked on food, boil baking soda and water in the pan for a few minutes. Scrub out with kitchen netting or a pot scrubber.

Grease spots left on pots and pans can be removed by rubbing the area with a little baking soda and rinsing clean.

Stainless steel cookware can be made to look like new again. Scrub aged pots and pans using baking soda with a sponge dampened with just a touch of vinegar. Buff to a shine.

Scorched pans can be made clean again by boiling 2 cups of water and a scant 1/4 cup of baking soda in pan. Let stand overnight and wash clean with dish detergent in the morning.

Baking soda and water can be used to clean and freshen the inside of lunch boxes. If seriously stained or if odors are intense, let the baking soda and water set in the container for at least an hour or two.

Spills and Stains
For quick wipe ups and spills, keep a spray bottle of environmentally responsible cleaner on hand. Mix 2 cups of water, 1 tablespoon baking soda and 3 tablespoons of vinegar.

For really difficult stains, add water to baking soda

to make a paste and let it dry on the dish. Rub off with a damp cloth for bright, revived dishes.

Coffee mug "rings" can be removed from countertops by rubbing down with a light soda paste. Just mix baking soda with a few tablespoons of water. Rub paste on the stain, let sit a few minutes and wipe away. For stubborn stains, rub with a baking soda containing toothpaste.

Ever spill something really sticky on your kitchen floor? Even honey wipes up easily with a cloth that has been wrung out of baking soda and water. Just scoop up what you can of the sticky mess and then wipe the remainder away with lots of water and baking soda. Clean up will be swift and all the stickiness will be gone.

Drains
To unclog a drain, mix 3/4 cup baking soda with 1 cup hot vinegar. Pour mixture down drain and let set for 5 minutes. Run very hot or boiling water down the drain to clear.

For tough clogs or drains clogged with grease, mix 3/4 cup baking soda, 3/4 cup salt and 1 cup hot vinegar. Pour the solution down the drain and let stand for one hour. Flush by running lots of very hot water down the drain.

BATHROOMS

Bathroom Fixtures
Baking soda is perfect for scrubbing bathroom fixtures without the danger of scratching shiny surfaces. Use on all sinks, tubs, shower stalls and toilets.

For gleaming brass surfaces, cover them with a

paste of baking soda and water. When dry, gently buff until they shine.

Remove rust stains from porcelain fixtures by wetting the stain with lemon juice and dusting generously with baking soda. When dry, re-wet and rub the stain away.

Bathtubs and Showers

To clean the greasy feel out of a bathtub after bathing with oils or gels, rub the tub down with baking soda as the water drains out.

Remove soap scum from shower doors by scrubbing them with baking soda. This is also good for removing soap build-up. Use on shower stalls, tubs and sinks.

Soak plastic shower curtains in hot water and baking soda to keep them from picking up mildew and mold.

Like to add oil to your bath, but hate the greasy clean up? Keep a box of baking soda handy and rub the tub down as the water drains out. No need to worry about getting harsh chemicals on your skin.

Tile and Grout

Use baking soda and water mixture to safely clean ceramic tile or marble floors.

Rub a paste of soda and vinegar over grout and let it dry. Wipe down with a cloth dampened in vinegar and it will look new again.

Toilet Cleaning

Dampen the toilet bowl and sprinkle heavily with baking soda. This will deodorize the bowl and help keep the porcelain clean. For stubborn stains, let set for a few minutes and then add some bleach. Swish it all around and let it set again for an hour or so. Rinse it all off and enjoy your sparkling clean, sweet smelling fixture.

Sinks and Drains

For tough sink and drain odors, clean the sink with baking soda. Then, rinse 1/2 cup baking soda down the drain using hot water. Follow with 1 cup of vinegar poured down the drain to finish.

Keep plumbing lines clean and odor-free by rinsing baking soda down drains as part of your monthly chores. Vinegar can be added for extra cleaning.

Make Your Own Scouring Powder

Baking soda is nature's perfect scouring powder!

Make your own safe, mildly abrasive cleaning solution to keep on hand for tough stains. Combine 1 cup vinegar and 1/4 cup baking soda in a jar and shake or stir well before using. DO NOT PUT A LID on this mixture while it is fizzing! This mixture can also be used to deodorize and absorb tough odors.

Mirrors

Wipe mirrors with water that has a little baking soda and vinegar added to it.

LIVING AREAS

Furniture

Clean vinyl furniture with warm water and baking soda. This removes grease and dirt without dulling the finish.

Clean chrome chair and table legs with a bit of soda on a damp cloth.

To help resolve moisture problems beneath the sink cupboards or other areas of your home, place an open box of baking soda to control humidity and odor problems.

Carpet and Rugs

For soiled spots in carpet, shake baking soda over the affected area and let stand overnight. Vacuum the carpet and dirt. Grease and odors will be gone, leaving your carpet smelling fresh and clean. You may need to repeat for stubborn soils.

Add baking soda directly to your vacuum cleaner bag to add a fresh after-vacuum smell to your home. For a floral scent, add a few drops of your favorite perfume.

To give an overall freshness to your carpeted living areas, sprinkle a light layer of baking soda over carpet and rugs before vacuuming.

Someone vomit on your carpet? Quick – grab the baking soda. It will neutralize the stomach acids that can bleach out flooring or upholstery fabric. When it dries, everything will vacuum up nice and neatly...with no smell! (And no disgusting gooey clean up.)

Spots, Stains and Scuffs

Use soda to clean ink, markers and crayons from vinyl flooring; also removes them from woodwork. For a stronger solution, add vinegar.

Baking soda can be used to scrub scuff marks off linoleum or vinyl floors.

Because baking soda is non-abrasive, it can be used to safely remove marks on most painted walls.

Someone spill wine on your carpet?? Don't panic!

To clean up spilled wine or grape juice stains, blot up as much of the spill as you can with a paper towel. Quickly sprinkle a thick layer of baking soda over the stained area and let set for at least an hour. Vacuum clean.

Windows

Use a solution of water with a touch of baking soda and vinegar to clean windows.

Spread baking soda along basement windows and door edges to keep insects at bay.

Wipe the frames of wooden windows with a strong baking soda solution to discourage mold from forming. This is especially important during winter months when cold weather can cause water to condense on window frames and encourage the growth of ugly black mold.

Walls

You can remove child's marker and crayon "artwork" from painted walls with a damp sponge and baking soda. Just clean in a soft, circular motion and wipe dry. Be sure to feather the edges so as not to leave a cleaning mark.

Wallpaper can be safely cleaned by gently wiping with a damp cloth wet with a water and baking soda solution. Dry when finished.

Wall Holes

Fix small holes in the wall with a combination of baking soda and toothpaste. Just mix lots of baking soda into a big dab of toothpaste, push it into the hole and give it time to dry.

Closets and Drawers

Place baking soda sachets in closets and clothing drawers to keep odors at bay.

For closets where moths are a problem, simply add an open box of baking soda or sachet full of soda to the area. Moths will disappear.

Renew your baking soda sachets by occasionally putting them out in the bright sun for a few hours. It will kill any germs they have collected and dry the soda out so that its ability to absorb moisture is renewed.

Baby's Nursery and Play Area

Wipe down baby's living area, including changing table, playpen and high chair, with baking soda on a damp sponge or towel. This will both clean stains and disinfect baby's area.

Baking soda can be used to clean and deodorize baby bottles. Just put baking soda and hot water in a bottle and close the lid. Then shake until the bottle is clean and rinse well.

Keep a fresh sachet of baking soda near baby's diaper pail to help absorb any unpleasant odors. Occasionally add a dash of baking soda to the pail to directly neutralize the urine.

Plastic children's toys can be disinfected and scrubbed down with baking soda and water for a clean new look.

Baby spit-up on upholstery can be easily cleaned with baking soda. Wipe up as much as possible with a rag. Sprinkle some baking soda on the area and wipe with a damp cloth. This will clean up and protect from staining, as well as prevent lingering odors. If the spit-up area still has an odor after cleaning, repeat as necessary.

Computer Housings

Gentle baking soda is the perfect abrasive for cleaning plastic computer housings. Always use a cloth wrung out of baking soda water, do not sprinkle baking soda where it can drift into keyboards or other mechanical parts.

Aluminum Doors

Make aluminum storm doors gleam by covering them with a paste of baking soda and lemon juice and letting them dry in the sun. Wipe off with a damp cloth. This is also a good treatment for dirty aluminum windows.

Basement

Baking soda can be used in the basement, around pipe openings, to repel roaches from entering your home. Apply a generous layer of baking soda all around the foundation as an additional protection from creepy crawlies.

Keep an opened box or two of baking soda in your basement to absorb musty odors and dampness.

If you are not going to use an appliance, such as a washer or dryer for a lengthy time, place a box of baking soda inside it to prevent mold and odors from building up.

Mold or Mildew

Mold or mildew on basement walls and floors can be scrubbed clean. In a bucket of warm water, add 1/4 cup of baking soda and a little vinegar. Scrub the moldy or mildewed area clean with a damp rag. For trouble spots, add some baking soda directly to your sponge or rag and scour in a circular motion. Rinse clean and dry well.

LAUNDRY

As consumers, we go to great lengths – at oftentimes very great expense – to launder garments and linens. Just as with other household cleaning products, large corporations are spending billions of dollars to get their latest must-have product off the store shelf and into our pantry. Most if it at unnecessary expense! Some of these products include:

- Pretreaters

- Stain removers

- Laundry detergent (even different detergents for different colors!)

- Dryer sheets

- Fabric softeners

- Rinse fresheners

And each of those new cleaners means yet one more chemical our bodies are exposed to! The wondrous properties of baking soda can do it all...safely, naturally and for just pennies!

A Natural Laundry Detergent

Baking soda is a natural companion to laundry cleaning. Whether it is used on its own as a stain fighter or added to your favorite laundry detergent for deeper cleaning, baking soda can help make your laundry cleaner and fresher.

Fabric Softener and Dryer Freshener

For softer clothes, add a half cup of baking soda to laundry rinse water.

Sprinkle a light mist of baking soda in your dryer along with your bathroom or pool towels. Dry as normal for fresh smelling linens.

Allergic to strong scents and cleaners? Add baking soda to your rinse water for an unscented and irritation-free fabric softener.

Pre-wash Treatment

Add baking soda to pre-wash water to remove the odor of urine from diapers and sickroom laundry.

Baking soda can be added to pre-wash water to eliminate odors from heavily soiled laundry. It will also begin the cleaning process for greasy or oily stains on clothes.

Stain and Spot Remover

For fabric stains, sprinkle baking soda directly onto the stain and add vinegar to spot clean it. The dirt spot will immediately begin to bubble and then it will fade away.

Use a mixture of soda water to remove tough stains on clothing and towels.

To pretreat laundry stains, rub a baking soda paste mixed with a few tablespoons of vinegar into a tough stain area. Let set for ten minutes before washing as normal.

Rust Stains

Many stains, including rust, can be removed from fabric by wetting with lemon juice, sprinkling with baking soda and letting it dry in the sun. this process may need to be repeated several times for full spot removal.

Heavily Soiled Garments
Add baking soda to liquid laundry detergent for better cleaning of heavily soiled garments.

Perspiration Smell and Stains
Soak clothes reeking of perspiration in a sink with warm water and baking soda before washing.

For perspiration stains, rub a baking soda paste into the stain and allow it to set for one hour. Wash clothing as normal.

Collar Stains
For ring-around-the-collar, rub a paste made of baking soda and vinegar into shirt collars before placing them in the washing machine. This can even be done as the clothes are placed in the dirty clothes hamper.

Sour Smelling Dishcloths
Sour smelling dishcloths can be renewed by adding baking soda to your wash cycle. This is also a good practice to use when washing your cleaning rags

For dishcloths or rags that are extremely rancid or sour, soak overnight in water with dishwashing soap and a few tablespoons of baking soda. Wash it out clean and fresh in the morning!

Rid Laundry of That Bleachy Smell
Using baking soda along with bleach when washing clothes will cut down on that "bleachy" smell on your clean laundry.

Adding soda to bleached clothes will also help to prevent rashes caused by bleach residue that may be sometimes left in clothes.

Clean Your Iron

Keep your iron free of sticky starch build-up by rubbing it down with baking soda and a little water. Remove starch build-up with baking soda and lemon juice paste. Do not put baking soda inside a steam iron.

Gentle Enough for Baby Clothes

Clean baby's plastic bibs with baking soda and a little water. It is safe for baby and easy to use.

For heavily soiled cloth diapers, add 1 cup of baking soda to hot water and wash as usual.

To gently prewash new clothes for baby, wash in 1/2 cup of baking soda added to a mild detergent. Rinse clean.

Combine with Bleach to Disinfect

Combine baking soda with bleach for enhanced cleaning and disinfecting power.

STILL MORE USES

Baking soda's uses are seemingly endless! Try a few of the following to make household chores easier!

Christmas Decorations

Make Christmas decorations especially festive by adding a sprinkling of baking soda snow! It will soak up odors and sweep up easily.

Sprinkle baking soda on your fresh Christmas tree; it will add a wintery look.

Musical Instruments

Use baking soda to clean and disinfect musical instrument mouth pieces.

To bring a high shine back to brass instruments, coat instrument with a thin layer of paste made from baking soda and a little water. Allow to dry and then buff to a high shine with a soft cloth.

To clean yellowed piano keys back to new, mix 1 quart of warm water with 1/3 cup of baking soda in a bowl. Clean piano keys with a cloth dampened in solution and wipe dry.

Clean CDs

CD scratches can be removed with a gentle cleaning of baking soda and a touch of water. Wipe with a clean cloth to remove any residue when finished and dry completely before using. Never use baking soda to clean DVDs.

Polish Jewelry

Baking soda paste can be used to clean some kinds of jewelry back to a sparkling shine.

Silver tarnish will disappear and jewelry can be brought back to new by gently rubbing it with a baking soda paste made of 3 tablespoons of baking soda and a teaspoon of water. Rinse when finished and buff dry with a soft cloth.

Do NOT clean pearls with baking soda, since this can damage delicate pearls. Opals are also too soft to be cleaned with any abrasive, even one as mild as baking soda.

Deodorize Humidifiers

Add a few tablespoons of baking soda to the humidifier water each time you fill the unit. This will keep away any musty smell and freshen the air as it humidifies.

Clean Hot Rollers and Curling Irons

Clean sticky residue off hot rollers by letting a paste of baking soda and lemon juice dry on them. Then, rub the accumulated gunk off. Also works great on curling irons and flat irons.

Super dirty hot rollers may be cleaned with a paste made of equal parts baking soda, salt and lemon juice.

Musty Odor on Books and Magazines

Take musty books and magazines and place them individually in brown paper bags. Add a few tablespoons of baking soda and close the bag. Keep the bag closed for at least a week. Shake soda off of the magazine or book and it should be free of any musty odor.

Help to prevent musty odors in the first place by sprinkling a little baking soda on bookshelves before adding books.

Snow and Ice Melter

Sprinkle baking soda on walkways, driveways and doorsteps to deice. You can also sprinkle it around the driveway, like sand, to help with traction.

Clean and Deodorize Air-Filters

Vacuum off dust and dirt from air filters. Then wash them in a bucket of warm water with 1/4 cup of baking soda added to it. Dry each filter completely before returning it to its machine.

Attention Hunters!!

Add a cup or two of baking soda to your wash water before you wash hunting clothes. This will rid them of that "human smell" animals pick up on so easily.

When storing hunting clothes between seasons, seal them in a box or bag sprinkled with baking soda. This will prevent deer and other animals from picking up on your scent or other odors unfamiliar to them. And, it will help to keep them from developing a musty odor.

Don't forget to treat your hunting boots, as well. Wash the outside of hunting boots in a baking soda and warm water wash. Sprinkle soda inside boots to rid them of human odors. Your feet will also enjoy this treatment.

BAKING SODA EATS ODORS

Baking soda neutralizes odors, rather than just covering them up, unlike many store bought air fresheners. This is because most disagreeable odors come from strong acids or bases, such as sour milk and rotten fish. Baking soda can bring both of these to a more neutral state, thus eliminating the odor. Baking soda also boasts a wonderful absorbing effect that helps get rid of musty and mildew odors that most air fresheners cannot touch, leaving notoriously stinky spaces smelling fresh and clean again!

Pickle and Sauerkraut Odor

Clear the odor of pickles or sauerkraut from plastic storage containers by filling them with cool water and adding a teaspoon of baking soda.

Diaper Pails

Use baking soda in the bottom of diaper pails to help eliminate diaper odor.

Shoe Odor
Fill a couple of old socks with baking soda and use them to fill shoes between wearing to eliminate foot odor. Every few months, set the soda-filled socks in the sun for an hour or two to freshen them up once again.

Backpacks
Clean backpacks with baking soda and water to neutralize odors.

Smelly Dishwashers
Sprinkle a light coating of baking soda in the bottom of the dishwasher before cleaning dishes. This will help eliminate all odors from dishes. You may want to add a dash of bleach too. It will help to kill germs.

Smoke Damage
For smoke damage, wipe down the area with cool water and baking soda. It will neutralize the unpleasant smell.

Cigarette Smell
Cigarette odor can get trapped easily in fabrics such as carpets, upholstery and curtains. Just sprinkle some baking soda on the affected areas and let them stand for a few hours before vacuuming them clean.

Add a quarter cup of baking soda to the vacuum cleaner bag when cleaning any area where cigarette or cigar odors are a problem.

Carpet, Rugs and Upholstery
To deodorize carpet, shake baking soda over area and let stand overnight. Vacuum the carpet the following day and odors will be gone. You can also use half baking soda and half cornstarch.

Add a tablespoon of baking soda to each new vacuum cleaner bag. It will help soak up all kinds of troublesome household odors.

Help keep your home smelling fresh by sprinkling baking soda over the floor before laying under-carpet padding.

Make Your Own Carpet and Upholstery Deodorizer
Make your own carpet or upholstery deodorizer by placing 1 cup of baking soda into a plastic shaker can. Add in fresh, full leaf mint leaves (that won't pass thru the shaker). You can also combine your favorite scented talc or several drops of your favorite perfume with the baking soda for a personalized scent. Chopped lemon or orange rinds make a good addition, too.

Refrigerator and Freezer
To make your refrigerator and freezer odor free, cut the top panel off the box of baking soda and place the entire box in the refrigerator or freezer.

Keep Ice Cubes Fresh
Place an open box of soda in your refrigerator's freezer to keep ice cubes fresh and odor-free.

To make your in-the-refrigerator (or freezer) box of odor absorbing baking soda work even better, lay a cotton ball with a little vanilla dripped onto it on the top of the box.

To eliminate a rotten smell in the freezer, wipe it down with vanilla, baking soda and water. Freeze the rotten food, then bag and dispose of it.

Counter Spoiled Food Odors
Eliminate the odor of spoiled foods in your refrigerator

by wiping down the shelves with a strong mixture of baking soda and water. Repeat if necessary.

Sinks and Drains

Don't throw away that old box of baking soda! Once you have finished using baking soda to absorb odors in places like the refrigerator, freezer or dark storage spaces, rinse the used box of soda down the kitchen drain, adding only a little at a time. This will help freshen garbage disposals and smelly sink drains. Be sure to use lots of hot water, so that the baking soda does not fill the sink trap and stop up the drain.

Keep drains sweet smelling and eliminate the odor that builds up in drains that will not be used for a while, such as when you are on vacation. Add a couple of tablespoons of baking soda to the drain and let it stay there without adding extra water. When you return home, rinse it all away and enjoy your sweet smelling home.

Use water with a cup of baking soda dissolved in it to deodorize sinks, garbage disposals, tubs, shower stalls and toilets.

Be careful not to add too much soda to drains at one time. Too much can result in a solid mass of baking soda in the sink trap.

Make Your Own Room Deodorizer

Make your own room deodorizer by adding a few fresh mint leaves to a cup of baking soda. You can also use a few drops of vanilla, your favorite perfume or scented talc.

The next time you have a few leaves left over from your favorite cooking herb, try adding them to some baking soda and putting the mixture in your vacuum cleaner bag. You may be surprised at how much you like the unexpected smell your freshly cleaned rooms will have!

Vacation Homes and RVs

Dust floors and counters of your vacation home or beach house with baking soda when you close them up for the season to prevent musty smells.

Tuck small sachets of baking soda throughout RVs and camper trailers before closing them up for the season. Dust shelves and inside drawers with the soda. They will not be stale-smelling in the spring.

This will also help to discourage nasty crawling insects from making a home in your unused home or vehicle.

Standing Water

Odors associated with standing water in places like basement drains or overflows can be neutralized by pouring baking soda down the drain. You can even use the ready-to-be-discarded boxes of soda from your refrigerator or crawl space!

Picnic Coolers

Place a small box or sachet of baking soda inside a picnic cooler during storage to eliminate that musty smell.

And do not forget to add some baking soda to that big thermos jug you use for lemonade and iced tea in the summer. During winter storage it will collect musty odors and moldy yuck if it is not treated with a couple of dashes of baking powder.

Linens, Pillows and Towels

Put a teaspoon of baking soda inside the ticking of new pillows. It will help to keep them from picking up body odor.

Linens and towels will be fresher smelling if closet shelves are dusted with baking soda.

Use extra baking soda to rinse out towels kept in gym bags or school lockers. They need all the help they can get to stay fresh!

Closets, Attics and Basements

Tuck packets of baking soda into the corners of closets, attics, storage shelves, crawl spaces, kitchen cupboards and under sinks to prevent nasty smells.

Fight basement moisture by applying baking soda to the top of the foundation, where the basement walls meet the first floor flooring. This will also deter bugs and worms.

Sprinkle extra baking soda on attic floors and joists before adding new insulation. Be sure to cover all the outside edges with soda, as this is one of the spots most likely to collect moisture and so form mold or mildew.

Garbage Cans

A kitchen garbage can will be freshened up with baking soda between the plastic can and liner.

For garbage cans that hold that "garbage" smell even after the trash has been taken out, try this trick. Empty the garbage can and wash the inside and outside with a wet rag or sponge sprinkled with baking soda. Rinse clean and dry completely. Add some baking soda to the bottom of the newly deodorized trash can before putting in the fresh liner. Add a little baking soda each time you change liners and your can will remain odor free.

Garbage Disposals

Clean out the odor in your garbage disposal with a periodic rinsing with baking soda. Adding a few ice cubes to the soda will also help.

Make Your Own Freshener Sachet

A good way to make small baking soda sachets is to put a cup of it into the toe of an old panty hose, make a knot, move up three inches, make another knot, add another cup of soda, make two more knots and add more soda, and end with a knot. Then cut the hose between knots and you will have several sachets of just the right size to tuck away into corners of the home and garage... or anywhere that needs a fresh scent!

Storage Bags and Boxes

Add a sachet containing baking soda to boxes and bags of clothes you are storing to prevent mustiness. Include a few scented herb leaves in the soda for additional freshness.

A small bag or sachet of baking soda in a suitcase will keep it fresh between uses.

Leave the sachet in your packed suitcase to keep the clothes from picking up odors as you travel. It will also help to fight musty odors in damp climates or aboard ships.

Ashtrays

Put half an inch of baking soda in the bottom of ashtrays throughout the house to prevent unpleasant smells.

A layer of baking soda can also be placed in the bottom of ashtrays in cars. This is a neat way to keep the car smelling fresh, particularly for those who do not smoke.

Fish Tanks

Scrub the inside of fish tanks with baking soda to remove the fishy odor; also great for bird cages and terrariums. Use baking soda's mild abrasive power to scrub off the algae and other scum that can stick to the glass.

Pets

Add a thick layer of baking soda to the bottom of cat litter boxes to help prevent lingering odors.

Sports Equipment and Workouts

Wipe down treadmills, stationary bikes and other home workout equipment with baking soda, vinegar and water to prevent germ accumulation and odor build up.

Deodorize sports equipment such as gym and golf bags by sprinkling the inside of them with baking soda.

Keep an open box of baking soda in a workout room to help absorb odors and keep the room smelling fresh.

FIRE AND SAFETY

Baking soda can be used to help put out small electrical or grease fires in your home by smothering and extinguishing small flames. ***REMEMBER TO NEVER USE BAKING SODA MIXED WITH WATER ON ANY ELECTRICAL OR GREASE FIRE!*** Simply dump the box of baking soda on the small flame, or toss a fistful of baking soda from a safe distance. Be sure and call the fire department to be certain the fire has been completely extinguished! Once the fire has been put out, allow the baking soda and fire element to completely cool before placing in the trash. This will ensure the flame does not re-ignite!

Keep an open box of baking soda near the stove; it

is good for putting out fires, especially grease fires.

Put Out Grease Fires
Use DRY baking soda to put out grease fires.
NEVER use baking soda and WATER on an electrical fire.

Fireplaces
Don't forget to have a box of baking soda on hand near the fireplace. Spread soda on any sparks that fly out before they start a house fire.

Christmas Trees
Keep a dish of baking soda near the Christmas tree to dump on an electrical fire that a short in the lights might cause. Never put water on an electrical fire!!

Garages and Workshops
Have an extra box of baking soda close by in the garage or workshop for small electric or engine fires. Remember to NEVER use water on any electrical fire! Call your local fire department if there is any doubt the fire has been permanently extinguished.

Treat Icy Sidewalks
Need to quickly treat an icy sidewalk spot? Simply grab the baking soda and sprinkle it on. It works on snow and ice.

STOP! DON'T THROW OUT THAT OLD BOX OF SODA!

Not only is baking soda an inexpensive alternative, but did you know it can be used again and again?

Boxes of baking soda which have been used to absorb odors in areas like refrigerators, freezers, attics and crawl spaces eventually need to be changed. But, once these boxes have done their job and are ready to be replaced...don't throw them out! There are still plenty of uses left in these amazing boxes. Try old baking soda you are about to discard in these trouble areas:

Outdoor Garbage Cans

Freshen outdoor garbage and trash cans by pouring old baking soda between the trash can and its liner.

Compost Piles

Pour contents of a used box of soda over compost piles to cut down on lingering odors.

Garbage Disposals, Sinks and Drains

Rinse down garage or basement drains to kill stench.

Septic Tank

To help keep your septic tank working at its best, dump a used box of baking soda down the drain once a month. Be sure to pour a little at a time and use lots of water.

Toilet

Pour part of an old box of soda into the toilet and let set for 20 minutes. Flush it away to help rinse out germs and leave the bowl smelling fresh. Do not use the entire box at one time, as soda can collect in the trap and plug the drain.

Standing Yard Water

Sprinkle on top of standing puddles in the yard to keep bugs from nesting.

Pour over yard puddles to eliminate mildew stench.

Tomato Plants

Empty an old box of baking soda around tomato plants in your vegetable garden to reduce the acidity of tomatoes.

Rain Gutters

Dump a discarded box of soda into easy-to-reach rain gutters and flush clean with a garden hose. This will help cut odors brewing in gutters and downspouts.

Pet Spots

Empty boxes of baking soda that are about to be thrown away over dog's "personal" area of his yard to absorb urine and feces odor. Unlike many commercial products, baking soda will not damage grass or landscaping!

Sprinkle extra baking soda over outdoor dogs' sleeping areas and inside dog houses to help get rid of doggy odor.

Chapter Three

OUTDOOR USES

It is well established that baking soda boasts a multitude of uses in keeping our homes clean and odor-free. But, let's not limit baking soda's use to just the inside of our homes. There are endless uses outside our doors to conquer everything from grease and grime in garages to eliminating unwanted pests and bugs and landscaping dilemmas. Baking soda can even help neutralize pH levels in swimming pools and ponds!

So, while we have already tackled indoor uses for this amazing mineral, let's head outdoors for more incredible uses.

GARAGES, PATIOS AND DECKS

Garages, patios, decks and other outdoor living spaces present their own, unique cleaning and care requirements. These high-maintenance areas easily get dirty and are subject to the ever-changing elements of weather. Remember to keep a box or two of baking soda on hand for these often overlooked areas.

Engine Fires
Keep a spare box of baking soda on hand for small electrical or engine fires. Remember to

NEVER use baking soda (or any material) mixed with water for an electrical fire!

Windows

Dirty window shutters can easily be cleaned with a baking soda and vinegar spray. Just spray shutters and let set for about 20 minutes. Wipe any tough areas and spray with a garden hose to rinse clean.

Clean outdoor window screens with 1/2 cup of baking soda and 1 cup of vinegar mixed into a bucket of water. Gently scrub screens with a soft brush and rinse clean with a garden hose.

Grease and Oil

Automobile grease can easily be cleaned up with baking soda and warm water solution.

Degrease lawn mowers and tractors with straight baking soda.

Oil drips in driveways can be cleaned up by pouring on a thick layer of baking soda. Allow it to set until the residue has soaked into the soda and then scoop it all up. Finish off by cleaning the area with baking soda and water.

Hand Tools

Clean hand tools periodically by wiping down with a damp rag and baking soda.

Garage Walls

Dingy garage walls can be whitened with a combination of baking soda and bleach. The baking soda will act as a mild abrasive and enhance the cleaning and whitening power of bleach.

Rust Stains

Rust stains can be scoured away with a solution of baking soda and vinegar.

Battery Acid

Neutralize any battery acid spills with baking soda.

Moss

Try sprinkling baking soda to rid unwanted moss on patios, walkways and garden paths. Also works great removing moss growing in cracks in concrete driveways and walks.

Lawn Fungus

Prevent unsightly lawn fungus with this natural solution. Mix 1/4 cup baking soda with 1/4 cup vegetable oil. Add 1 teaspoon of dishwashing soap. Combine all ingredients in a gallon jug of water. Spray on lawn to prevent fungus from growing. Great for shaded areas of your lawn, too.

Tree Sap

Clean tree sap off your deck by rubbing with baking soda and warm water.

Outdoor Grill

Stains from your outdoor grill and cooking can be removed by covering them with baking soda and letting it stand for an hour or so. Wipe clean and rinse well.

After cooking, wash outdoor grills with baking soda and vinegar. The job will be much easier if you do it while they are still warm.

Remove baked-on or burned foods from outdoor grills. Remove grill plate from unit. Soak in a heavy mixture of 1 cup baking soda and 1 cup of vinegar for two hours.

Clean with a hard bristle brush and rinse. Dry with a towel to prevent rusting.

Deck and Patio Furniture

Plastic deck furniture and vinyl chairs can look beautiful again after being cleaned with a baking soda paste. This is a great deck furniture cleaner for both beginning and end-of-season clean up.

Clean lawn furniture without scratching metals or plastic by wiping with a baking soda and a wet sponge.

Patio umbrellas can be cleaned of smelly mildew and mold by being washed with a solution of 1 cup baking soda and a half bucket of warm water. Open umbrella and allow it to dry in the open sunshine. Sprinkle it, inside and out, with baking soda before storing it away for the season and it will not collect mold over the winter.

Outdoor resin furniture can be made like new again with a light baking soda and warm water scrubbing. Put soda on a damp sponge and apply in a circular motion. Rinse in clear, warm water and allow to air dry in the sunshine.

Mold and Mildew

Mildew on outdoor decks can be eliminated by spraying with mixture of baking soda and water or vinegar. Let the mixture stand on the deck for a few minutes, them use a stiff broom to brush away the mildew. Rinse and apply a second coating that does not need to be rinsed off.

Pool Toys

Pool toys can be disinfected by washing them in 1/3 cup of baking soda and a quart of warm water. Also kills mildew and prevents mold form easily forming.

Bird Baths and Feeders

Occasionally rinse and clean bird baths with baking soda and water to keep germs and algae from growing.

Bird and animal feeders can be safely cleaned with a baking soda and water rinse.

AUTOMOBILES AND RECREATIONAL VEHICLES

Baking soda, while wonderful at cleaning and disinfecting, is also a mild abrasive safe for glass, plastic, fiberglass and chrome. Don't forget about using baking soda as an effective cleaner for the inside and outside of your cars, trucks and recreational vehicles.

Windshields

Wipe windshield washers clean with baking soda and a damp sponge or cloth. Rinse clean.

To use as a rain repellent on your windshield, simply wipe baking soda across windshield with a damp cloth.

Bugs on your windshield or bumper can be easily removed with baking soda and a scrubbing cloth.

Wipe windshields, windows and mirrors with water that has a little baking soda and vinegar added to it and greasy smears will disappear.

Use a baking soda and water mixture to wash car windows. It will remove the haze that builds up on windshields when the salt that is used on icy roads is splashed onto them.

Cut Down on Streaks and Glare

For no streak window cleaning, pat a paste of soda and water onto the glass and let dry. Buff off with a soft, dry cloth.

Chrome

Renew old chrome by coating with a thin paste made from baking soda and water. Allow to dry and then buff to a high shine with a soft cloth.

Clean chrome car trim, bumpers and wheels with baking soda and water or vinegar.

Automobile Grease or Tar

Tree sap or tar on your automobile can be rubbed off with a soft solution of baking soda and a wet sponge or car cloth.

Greasy Garage Hands

Hands greasy from working on your brakes or engine? Wash with baking soda and warm water to remove the greasy grime.

Grease Stains on Garage Floors

Grease stains on garage floors can be eliminated by washing with baking soda and water.

Difficult stains on your concrete garage floor can be removed with a heavier concentration of baking soda and warm water. Lightly spray soiled area with a garden hose and sprinkle a heavy layer of baking soda over the entire affected area. Let set undisturbed for 10 minutes. Pour a small amount of hot water over the treated area and scrub with a wire brush.

Neutralize Battery Acid

Car battery acid can be neutralized by covering with

baking soda. With gloves, carefully scoop up the acid after it has been fully absorbed.

Battery acid that has been on terminals for a long time can be removed by scrubbing the terminals with an old toothbrush and baking soda. Be sure to rinse is all off.

Ashtrays
Sprinkle a thick layer of baking soda in the bottom of your car's ashtray to help absorb odors in the entire car. Add a couple of mint leaves to each unused ashtray for an especially clean smell.

Carpets and Floor Mats
Carpets and cloth floor mats can be deodorized by sprinkling with baking soda before vacuuming.

Scuffs and Scratches
Scuffs and scratches on your automobiles dashboard can be muted by buffing out with baking soda and water.

Eliminate Musty RV Smell
Set an open box of baking soda on a counter in your RV or camper to prevent musty smells from building up.

Campers and RVs are small, enclosed areas where musty smells can build up very quickly. Consider making a baking soda air freshener. In a pretty bowl or jar, add 1/2 cup of baking soda mixed with your favorite talc or perfume. Place fresheners around your recreational vehicle to keep it smelling fresh all day. Leave the air fresheners in the vehicle during storage.

Freshwater Holding Tanks
Once each season, rinse out the fresh water holding tank of boats or recreational vehicles with baking soda.

Mineral Deposits
For removing mineral deposits and keeping your freshwater RV tank clean, flush with a cup of baking soda dissolved in 1 gallon of warm water once or twice a season. Flush out baking soda water before filling with fresh drinking water.

Bilges
Every season, dump a little baking soda into bilge areas in boats or RVs. Let set a few hours and pump out.

RV Toilets
Controlling odor in recreation vehicle toilets is simple. Just pour a box of baking soda into your holding tank after it has been emptied.

RV Winter Storage
Before closing up your RV for winter storage, place boxes or sachets of baking soda throughout (including inside drawers and cupboards). You can even sprinkle baking soda on the floors and countertops. This will eliminate that mildew smell in the spring! It will also discourage crawling insects from making your vehicle their home.

Camper Shower Stalls
Use baking soda and vinegar to wash the insides of shower stalls to leave your camper smelling fresh and clean.

POOLS, PONDS AND AQUARIUMS

The success of pools, ponds and aquariums depends heavily on pH balance. Did you know baking soda is one of the best natural neutralizers of pH levels?

Simply put, pH is the measuring of how much acid

or alkaline can be found in something such as garden soil or pond water. Ecosystems, plant and wildlife all depend heavily on balanced pH levels. The pH measurement scale runs from 1 to 14, with the lower end (1) being extremely acidic and the higher end (14) being extremely alkaline. How effective you are at maintaining a healthy pH level in your pond or garden will be evident in healthy plants and thriving pond life.

For example, there are fluctuations in pH levels between night and day due to photosynthesis activity in plants...which can kill fish.

In addition, some flowering plants, such as begonias or geraniums, thrive in a pH soil level of 5. Koi ponds demand a pH between 7 and 9, while swimming pool water needs to be in the mid 7s.

Baking soda can help adjust these pH levels naturally and without harmful chemical additives. This translates to livelier vegetable and flower gardens and a healthier environment in pools and ponds. Adjusting the pH level in swimming pools means clearer water and less harsh chemicals that can dry out and irritate sensitive skin.

For some natural ways to enhance your pools, ponds and aquariums, try a few of these simple solutions.

Adjusting pH Levels in Pools and Ponds
To adjust the pH level in swimming pools without the use of chlorine, add one and a half pounds of baking soda to each 10,000 gallons of water.

For ponds, use a cup of baking soda for each 500 gallons of water to bring water to a more neutral and acceptable pH level.

Use about a tablespoon of baking soda for every 10 gallons of pond water to stabilize and balance pH levels. You can use this same solution for large aquariums without the risk of harming fish.

Cleaning Slip and Slime from Pool Walkways
To clean off pool walkways and tile, sprinkle heavily with baking soda and use a mop to wipe clean. Simply rinse away.

Use baking soda and water in a spray bottle to clean slippery scum off rocks surrounding the edges of your koi pond.

Pool Toys
Children's pool toys can safely be cleaned by washing in warm water and baking soda.

Pool Tools
Clean the muck and grime from pool nets and lines by washing in a bucket of warm water mixed with baking soda and a little bleach.

Pool Floats and Toys
Scrub plastic pool floats and toys with a solution of water and baking soda to remove any film that builds up.

Child's Pool
Put a handful of baking soda in the water of your child's plastic pool to keep the water clean and clear of bacteria and soothe your child's skin.

Moldy Pool Toys
To remove and disinfect plastic pool toys that have picked up mold or mildew, rub down area with a baking soda paste made from 3 – 4 tablespoons of baking soda and a tablespoon of water. You can also add a touch of

bleach for any heavily soiled or smelly items.

Aquariums and Terrariums

Try adding 1 teaspoon of baking soda to every 5 gallons of aquarium water in your fish tank to keep your pH level balanced and the water smelling fresh and clear.

Baking soda is a natural solution to combat both fungus and bacteria in fish tanks. Add 2 teaspoons to a 10 gallon aquarium to keep your fish healthy and happy.

You can clean aquarium decorations and ornamental plastic grasses with baking soda and water. Simply rinse when finished and replace. Do not worry if some of the excess baking soda goes back into the tank... remember, baking soda is good for maintaining a healthy balance between alkaline and acidity levels in the fish's environment.

Baking soda works great as a safe glass cleaner for fish tanks.

Clean scum and buildup off fish nets and supplies by soaking in baking soda and warm water.

Remove Algae from Fountains

Algae build up on outdoor fountains can be banished with a light cleaning of baking soda and warm water. Use a brush to remove heavy algae growths.

Adding a few tablespoons of baking soda to your fountain water can help cut down on algae build up and slime.

Fountain Pumps

Water fountain pumps can also be cleaned with baking soda. It can be used to remove scummy residue and build up for more efficient pumping action.

Chapter Four

PETS, PESTS AND PLANTS

Baking soda is widely known for its multitude of uses as a natural household cleaning agent. Its unique properties make it not only a versatile deep cleaner without unwanted harsh chemical compounds, but also an inexpensive alternative to expensive store bought cleaners. It boasts non-abrasive cleaning qualities that will not damage porcelain or fine china.

But, the use of baking soda and a cleaner should not be limited to indoors only. Its use outdoors is just as unlimited! A mineral that occurs naturally makes it the perfect companion to gardening, animal and pet care, and even a natural pesticide. If you are considering going "green," go green with baking soda!

One of the most overlooked properties of baking soda is its ability to regulate pH balance in everything from water to soil. When added to garden or landscaping soil, it works to neutralize high pH levels and eliminate strong acidity which can be detrimental to garden crops. Equalizing pH levels in water can also make laundry water less harsh. It can be used as an anti-fungal and even rid your vegetable garden of boring insects...making it the perfect, natural garden companion!

And because baking soda is safe to eat, it makes a wonderful addition to your pet's bathing routine.

Once you begin incorporating baking soda into your gardening and landscaping routine, you will soon be able to reap countless benefits of this mineral's unique properties. Try baking soda in the garden, on the patio, in the garage...anywhere a natural alternative is needed!

PETS

Don't forget that pets can benefit from wonderful baking soda, too!

Because natural baking soda is safe to eat, it makes the perfect accompaniment to keeping your pets clean and fresh. Just make sure your pet does not eat too much of it. Unlike harsh chemicals that leave your pet's skin dry and irritated, baking soda is a mild agent that soothes skin, absorbs odors and keeps your pet's coat soft and clean. And, you can use it every day, if necessary.

Hair and Fur
Keep your dog's fur clean and odor-free between baths by brushing a few tablespoons of baking soda through his fur. This will not only eliminate odor between baths, but also leave his hair shiny and healthy. Also works on cats, rabbits, ferrets, mice, gerbils, hamsters, guinea pigs and chinchillas.

Add a little baking soda to dog shampoo for odor control.

For a quick "dry bath" when there is no time to shampoo, comb some baking soda through your dog's fur to give him a quick clean and leave him smelling fresh and odor-free.

After bathing the dog in its usual shampoo, finish off with a water and baking soda leave in rinse to help control itching.

Litter Boxes

Sprinkle a thick layer of baking soda in the container before adding cat litter; you will have fewer odor problems.

Make your own kitty litter. Combine 1 box of baking soda with 3 – 4 inches of dry clay in your litter pan. Mix together.

Teeth and Breath

Keep your pet's teeth clean by brushing them with baking soda. Wet a soft cloth and use it to cover a finger. Then dip the tip of your finger into baking soda and use your finger to brush the pet's teeth. You can also use a special animal toothbrush.

For bad doggie breath, spray dog's mouth with a simple solution mixed from 1 cup water and 1/2 teaspoon of baking soda.

Your dog's teeth can be brushed with baking soda to keep tartar under control. Dog toothbrushes are available from pet stores, or simply use a soft-bristled toothbrush. Remember to brush your dog's teeth gently, getting between the teeth. Rinse with cool water.

Ear Wash

For dogs and cats that are scratching their ears, give them some gentle relief with this solution. Wet a cotton ball or tissue in warm water and dip in baking soda. Gently rub inside of your pet's ears to relieve the itching.

Baths and Washes

Put two cups of baking soda in the dog's bath water to keep him from developing doggie odor...especially when he's wet!

To keep your dog's coat shiny, add 2 tablespoons of baking soda to his bath water when rinsing.

Accidents and Stains

Rub baking soda into carpet where a dog has had an accident. When dry, vacuum up the odor.

For tough accident stains, sprinkle baking soda over the area and allow it to set. Scrub with a wet sponge or cleaning brush.

Baking soda can keep your puppy from returning to the same "accident" spot while potty training him. After cleaning up the dog's accident, sprinkle baking soda over the cleaned area to dilute the scent that makes puppy return.

Absorb Pet Odors

Want a great deodorizer for your pet? Dip a cat or dog's comb into baking soda and brush thru the pet's dry hair. This will keep pet odor from becoming a problem.

Rub baking soda into dog's belly to keep him smelling fresh and clean in between baths. This will also reduce the amount of scratching the dog does, as it soothes the skin to reduce itching.

To clean and disinfect your pet's travel crate, wash the crate on the inside and out with warm water and baking soda.

Add 1/2 cup of baking soda to your washing machine

when washing dog and cat beds to make them come out smelling fresh and clean.

Sprinkle baking soda over the area where your pet often lays. Allow to sit for several minutes and then vacuum. This will eliminate pet-smell in your home.

To freshen your pet's bedding area in between washings, sprinkle with baking soda and let set for 10 – 15 minutes. Vacuum.

If you're dog is sprayed by a skunk, hydrogen peroxide (3%) and baking soda can be mixed along with dog's regular wash to neutralize the unpleasant odor. Rinse well. After the dog is dry, rub baking soda into his fur to eliminate any lingering odor that may remain.

Use baking soda and water to scrub the inside of a dirty bird cage. This will clean the cage and eliminate unpleasant odor.

Ferret cages can be cleaned with baking soda and water. To continue controlling ferret odor, put a thin layer of baking soda in the cage beneath his bedding. This will help keep odors under control between bedding changes.

Toenails
If you happen to nick your dog's toe while trimming his nails, dip the nicked toe into baking soda and add pressure until the bleeding stops.

Protect Dog Dishes from Insects
To stop creepy crawlies from getting into your outdoor pet's food dish, pour a thick circle of baking soda around the pet's food dish. This will act as a barrier to keep bugs from crawling into the food dish for a nibble.

Stings and Insect Bites

To sooth your pet after it has been stung by a bee or wasp, carefully remove the stinger and coat the area with a thick paste made of baking soda and a little water.

For insect bites, wash the affected area, dry and coat with a thick baking soda paste.

To take the sting or pain out of insect bites, wrap a vinegar and baking soda poultice around affected area.

Cages, Crates and Toys

Pet toys from all types of animals can be cleaned and disinfected with baking soda and hot water.

Keep small animal cages clean by scrubbing with a solution of 1/3 cup of baking soda mixed into a quart of warm water. Scrub bottom and sides of cage and rinse clean. Dry with a towel. Sprinkle a thin layer of baking soda into the cage and place new bedding material on top of soda layer.

Baking soda is great for cleaning all tools and materials that come in contact with your salt water aquarium.

Fleas

Sprinkle a heavy layer of baking soda on carpet to kill fleas. Do this frequently during warm weather if you have a pet that spend much time outside during the day.

Fish and Aquariums

Scrub the inside of fish tanks with vinegar to remove scum and algae. Then scrub with baking soda to remove the fishy odor without scratching the aquarium glass and to neutralize the acid in vinegar. This double cleaning also works well for bird cages and terrariums.

PLANTS AND GARDENS

The secret to beautiful, bountiful flowerbeds and vegetable gardens can be found in good soil and tender care...a perfect match for the properties of baking soda!! Shelves at nurseries and garden centers are filled with every chemical and cure-all imaginable to combat all the woes of gardening.

- Harmful pests and boring insects

- Fungus

- Acidic soil levels

- Extreme alkaline soils

- Pesticides

- Compost odors

- Crabgrass and moss build up

- Animal repellents

- Ant and roach repellent

But these "cures" come with a price. Not just in the form of high monetary cost, but exposure to harmful chemicals and their long term residual effects on our bodies and nature itself. Do you really feel comfortable eating vegetables from your garden after using harsh chemicals? Science is still studying some of the long lasting effects from the use of these compounds, and no one knows for sure what the lasting effect will be on the environment.

- Do you struggle with aphids and other creepy crawlies dining on your garden vegetables, but are hesitant to use harmful pesticides on food your family eats?

- Tired of rabbits and other furry critters grazing in your garden, but are looking for a friendly way to shoo them away without harm?

- Have a problem with fungus or mildew growing on plant leaves, but unsure of using harsh chemical treatments?

Store bought treatments and commercial pesticides can bring unwanted exposure to chemicals with unknown long-term effects on both your health and the environment.

Baking soda, however, is 100% natural and safe enough for human consumption! We cook with it, clean with it, and even bathe in it. Baking soda is even known to help stimulate some vegetable growth! And, it is both child and pet-safe! From controlling pH levels and repelling harmful insects to keeping mold and fungus at bay and stimulating plant growth, baking soda does it all...for just a fraction of the price of dangerous poisons!

The next time you are thinking of reaching for a store bought, commercial garden product, consider trying one of these natural solutions instead!

Adjust Your Decorative Pond's pH Level
Adjust the pH level of your outdoor pond. Ponds have wide swings in pH levels from daytime to nighttime due to photosynthesis activity plants. This fluctuation can kill fish living in the ponds.

Use 1 cup of baking soda for each 500 gallons of water to bring your pond to a more neutral pH.

Mildew and Fungus

Baking soda can be used to control powdery mildew and other fungal diseases that attack garden plants. Use on roses, cucumbers, eggplant, strawberries, some melons, potatoes, wheat, peanuts, bananas, grapes and alfalfa.

Baking soda can be mixed with dish washing detergent to help deter fungus on rose bushes. Simply mix 1 tablespoon of soda in a gallon of water with a few drops of dish detergent. Gently spray on rose bushes.

Concerned about powdery mildew on plants? Use baking soda to control mildew and other fungal diseases that attack garden plants. Great for roses, cucumbers, eggplant, strawberries, some melons, potatoes, wheat, peanuts, bananas, grapes and alfalfa.

Plant mildew can be kept at bay with this mixture. Fill a clean spray container with 1 tablespoon of baking soda, 1/2 teaspoon of mild dish detergent and 1 gallon of water. Spray plants down with a garden hose to fully saturate with water (this will help protect the plants themselves). Once plants are wet, spray baking soda mixture directly onto plant leaves sparingly. Grapes, in particular, need to be sprayed on a regular basis.

Rid Yard of Mushrooms

Sprinkle lawn mushrooms with baking soda to make them go away.

Make Your Own "Sprinkle Shaker"

Make a baking soda "sprinkle shaker" to easily spread baking soda around tender plants and vegetables.

Take an empty carpet cleaner shaker and refill with baking soda. The light fall of baking soda will be easy to control in your garden and gentle on leaves and stems of delicate plants.

Yard Mold
Kill mold growing in yards and around your garden by spraying with a jug full of water treated with 1/4 cup of baking soda and a few tablespoons of bleach.

Garden Slugs
Baking soda is the perfect answer to combat garden slugs.

Pour around plants slugs are attracted to. Or, dust directly on plant leaves and slugs to eliminate these slippery creatures.

Sprinkling baking soda on cabbage and lettuce plants will keep slugs from devouring these plants. You can also make a circle around the plants with baking soda. Many pests will not crawl through it, especially the slimy ones.

Healthy Potting Soil
Add a layer of baking soda to the bottom of a pot before you add dirt and plants. This will keep the potting soil healthy and fresh for maximum growth.

Flowers
Apply a very small amount of baking soda to soil of flowers such as petunias and carnations.

Make Your Own Plant Food
Alkaline loving flowers, such as clematis and geraniums, thrive on this natural plant food. Just mix 1-2 tablespoons of baking soda in 2 quarts of water. Gently water flowers

for healthier plants.

Reduce Acidity in Tomatoes
Sprinkle baking soda on the soil around your tomato plants and gently work it into the soil. This will reduce the tomatoes acid content for sweeter, more delicious tomatoes!

Ants
Ants and other boring insects will stay away from your garden if you sprinkle liberal amounts of baking soda around the soil.

Pour baking soda around areas of your garden attacked by ants and other insects. The baking soda line will act as a barrier to crawling insects.

Compost Pile
Dump an old, used box of baking soda in your compost pile to keep the acidity level down.

Moss
Prevent moss from taking over your flower garden's walkway by sprinkling baking soda over the area.

Bunnies Nibbling??
Use baking soda around your vegetable garden to keep bunnies from nibbling.

Pesticide
A natural pesticide can be made by mixing 1/4 cup of vegetable oil and 1 teaspoon of baking soda together. After baking soda is fully dissolved, mix 1 tablespoon of this concoction into a cup of water. Fill a clean spray container and squirt directly onto plants. Great for deterring those pesky aphids and spider mites.

Cut Flowers

For cut flowers, add 1 tablespoon of baking soda to your flower's vase and fill with warm water to lengthen bloom life. Change the water everyday for the best results.

PESKY PESTS

Ick! Pesky pests can come in all shapes, forms and sizes. Not only are they pests and disgusting to have creeping and crawling through our homes and outdoor living area, but they can also spread sickness and disease.

Even the cleanest of homes may have trouble with these critters.

- Ants entering thru pipes and drain lines

- Cockroaches

- Nuisance ants

- Silverfish in the basement bathroom

- Aphids in the vegetable garden

- Centipedes

- Rodents

- Gnats ruining your picnic or barbeque

- Rabbits in your garden

Do you really want to use harmful chemicals in the areas of your home where you eat and sleep? Spray dangerous pesticides on the vegetables you eat? Leave bait traps out in the open where small children may find them?

And, what about extermination companies? Many of these companies specialize in ridding homes of unwanted insects by spraying chemical solutions used as a "barrier" around the perimeter of your home…both inside and outside. But what about the chemical residue that is left behind? Most extermination or preventative "treatments" must be repeated on a monthly basis to ensure bugs won't enter your home.

If you are not comfortable with chemical insecticides being sprayed on the living areas of your home, where small children and pets romp and play, maybe it's time to look for a better way!

Let's use a better, safer way … the natural way … through the amazing powers of wonderful baking soda!

Cockroaches
You can keep cockroaches from your kitchens and baths by sprinkling baking soda in cupboards and closets.

Make Your Own Bait Trap
Take a small container with a tight fitting lid, such as a margarine or cream cheese tub, and clean. Poke several very small holes in the side of the tub, just small enough for cockroaches to enter, but no larger. Mix 1 tablespoon of baking soda with 1 tablespoon of sugar and pour it into the container. Make sure the lid is on tight and place it in area cockroaches have been seen. Roaches will eat the solution and as their bellies swell, they become trapped inside. Great for spiders, earwigs and even cockroaches!

Ants
Pour baking soda around areas of your kitchen

where ants and other insects are attracted. The baking soda will act as a barrier to these crawling insects.

Ant problem in your basement or attic? Mix 1/4 cup of white vinegar with a few tablespoons of baking soda in an empty spray bottle. Fill with tap water. Spray trouble areas to get rid of ants.

Another way to repel ants is to mix crushed hot chilies with baking soda and spread the mixture along areas frequented by ants. It will upset their usual pathways and drive them away from your home.

Silverfish

Silverfish can be kept away by sprinkling baking soda in dark, damp areas of your home or storage places that can be havens for these small, but ghastly, creatures. Not only are they repulsive, they attract the centipedes, earwigs and spiders that feed on them.

Bait traps, such as the one recommended for cockroaches, can also be used for silverfish. Carefully poke holes in a small, plastic container no bigger than a silverfish can crawl through. Fill the container with baking soda and confectioner's (powdered) sugar and tightly close the lid. Place your trap in areas where silverfish have gathered. They will crawl inside, and after eating the bait, their bellies swell so they are unable to crawl back out the holes. Empty traps frequently.

Centipedes

Use baking soda throughout damp areas of your home to reduce moisture where these ugly creatures thrive. Keep an open box of soda in basements and sprinkle soda on carpets 30 minutes before vacuuming. This will help eliminate moisture and dampness that attract these bugs.

Natural Exterminator and Insecticide

Why pay for an exterminator to spray your home with toxic chemicals? To keep ants from entering or returning to your home, spray a vinegar and baking soda solution around the interior perimeter of your home. You may need to repeat once a month during the summertime or in warmer geographical areas. This natural pesticide is safe for both pets and small children.

Ant Hills

Find an ant colony taking up residence in your backyard? Spray the ant hill with enough water to saturate the hill. Pour about 2 cups of baking soda over the hill and let stand for about 20 minutes. Pour a cup of white vinegar over the hill and the baking soda, until a bubbling action takes place. The ant colony will be destroyed. Rain will merely wash more of the baking soda down into the old ant hill.

Rabbits in the Garden

Dump lots of baking soda around your garden to discourage bunnies from nibbling on your prized plants.

Gnats

Spray areas of your yard with a spray bottle filled with water and baking soda to rid the area of irritating gnats.

Chapter Five

LET'S GET PERSONAL: FROM THE INSIDE, OUT

Up to now, we have focused on baking soda as a wonderful, natural cleaning alternative and amazing absorber of all types of odors. It kills bacteria and fungi, freshens and deodorizes, neutralizes and balances pH levels. We have also used baking soda as a natural replacement for harsh chemicals and pesticides.

Now, it's time to get personal! Consider just a few of the products filling our medicine cabinets and drawers:

• Beauty regimen products

• Skin creams

• Deodorants

• Dental hygiene products

• Antacids

• Talcs and perfumes

• Toothpastes and washes

• Over the counter medications for small ailments

such as bladder infections

- Foot creams and soaks

- Bath beads, gels and soaks

...and the list could go on and on!

We all want to look and feel our best. But how much of what we buy do we really need? How much of what we buy really works? How many of the products on drug store shelves live up to their magnificent claims? How much of it is just fluff and empty promises?

Most importantly, ask yourself this question: Is there a better, safer and more natural way to take care of our bodies?

We have an old fashioned personal care product that is natural and costs just pennies in our own kitchen cupboard.

Sodium bicarbonate, or baking soda, is a fine powder that makes it perfect for all types of health and beauty uses. And, it is inexpensive enough to use for all our health and beauty needs. Just a few of baking soda's wondrous properties include:

- Baking soda is safe enough to ingest.

- It is a mild abrasive making the perfect natural facial scrub or skin exfoliator

- A wonderful absorbing agent that works against odors

- Soft, gentle powder is non-irritating to sensitive skin

- Soothing element can be used as a remedy for skin ailments

- And, it is completely natural!

Make it part of your cleaning routine ... in and out!

INSIDE THE BODY

So, are you ready to begin feeling better, the natural way? Welcome to the healing wonders of baking soda.

It is no surprise that many individuals have relied on the healing power of baking soda to cure all sorts of physical ailments for generations. Traditional medical systems focus on pharmaceuticals and invasive office procedures, all at a premium price! Many of us are returning to an old-time trusted friend in baking soda.

The idea of using baking soda for medicinal purposes is not a new concept! Not only has it been around for hundreds of years to treat every ailment from bee stings and insect bites to bladder infections and respiratory problems, but even modern day drug manufacturers have jumped on board. They are now spending millions of dollars per year to advertise what we already know... the use of baking soda (sometimes listed under the mineral name sodium bicarbonate) is now being used in their medications and health products.

Take a look at some of the packaging on a few of your favorite products in the drug aisle. Have you noticed how many products on our drug store shelves already tout the natural working power of baking soda?

Phrases like, "the whitening power of baking soda"

and "baking soda for a fresh and clean feeling" are everywhere.

Think about some of these products next time you are browsing the shelves in your local drug store:

- Toothpastes

- Mouthwash

- Yeast and itching medicines

- Antacids

- Heartburn tablets

- Bladder infection medications

So, it's no wonder baking soda is being hailed as a natural cure for so much of what ails us. Before you reach for that drug store medication, consider trying one of these baking soda home remedies…and treat your ailment the old-fashioned, natural way!

Remember, if you are on a salt-restricted diet, or have been advised by your physician to avoid sodium, do not take baking soda, as this could lead to serious health issues.

Allergies
Reduce allergy symptoms by sniffing up a mixture made with 1 cup of water, 1/3 teaspoon salt and a pinch of baking soda. Because there are no preservatives in this solution, you'll need to replace it every 24 hours.

Gas
Relieve gas in the stomach by sipping on a glass of

water to which a pinch of baking soda has been added.

End stomach gas pains by sipping on this concoction: a glass of water mixed with 2 tablespoons of lemon juice and 1/4 teaspoon of baking soda.

Stomach Acid
Relieve tummy pain from an acid stomach by sipping on a glass of water to which a pinch of soda has been added.

Heartburn
Relieve heartburn by sipping on a glass of water combined with a teaspoon of baking soda.

Indigestion
Eat something that just doesn't agree with you? Get rid of indigestion by drinking a small glass of water with a pinch of baking soda.

Acid Reflux
A concoction of apple cider vinegar and a teaspoon of baking soda mixed into a glass of water can help with the ails of acid reflux.

Calm an Upset Stomach
Slowly sip on a glass of lemon-lime soda with 1/2 teaspoon baking soda mixed in to ease the nauseated feeling of an upset stomach.

Mouth Ailments
End pains of mouth and canker sores with baking soda.

Cuts and sores on the inside of the mouth can be relieved by swishing mouth with a baking soda rinse. Just mix a few teaspoons of baking soda into a small glass of warm water. Use as a mouth rinse as often as necessary.

Bad Breath
Freshen breath with a gargle of baking soda and water.

Make your own gargle rinse using a cup of water and a teaspoon of baking soda.

Make Your Own Toothpaste
Sodium bicarbonate is found as an active ingredient in many commercial toothpastes and mouthwashes. You can make your own!

Make your own toothpaste by mixing a few drops of oil of peppermint in a small dish of baking soda. Just dip a wet toothbrush into the mixture and begin brushing.

Healthy Toothbrush Means Healthy Mouth
For a healthy mouth, dip toothbrush in hydrogen peroxide, then in baking soda. Soda neutralizes mouth acids before they can eat away at tooth surfaces and peroxide whitens teeth.

Clean and refresh your toothbrushes by soaking them overnight in a cup of warm water with a few table-spoons of baking soda added to it. Be sure to mix well.

Safely Whiten Teeth
As an alternative, dip toothbrush in equal parts baking soda and salt, and then into hydrogen peroxide for stronger neutralizing and whitening effect.

Dentures
Dentures can be cleaned and freshened by soaking in a glass of warm water and 1 tablespoon of baking soda. Let stand undisturbed for 20 – 30 minutes and then rinse

clean.

Retainers
Freshen dental retainers with a gentle combination of baking soda and water to stop odor.

Nose and Breathing
Add 1 – 2 tablespoons of baking soda to a humidifier. This will not only keep any musty smells at bay, but also keep bacteria from growing. Bacteria in the air can make breathing and allergy ailments worse.

Stuffy Nose
To relief stuffiness, rinse with a nasal solution of 1/2 cup of warm water, 1/4 teaspoon of baking soda and a pinch of salt. Repeat treatment as needed.

Gout
Take 1/2 teaspoon of baking soda daily with a meal to prevent gout.

Bladder Infections
Cystitis, a bladder infection that causes burning sensation during urination, can be soothed with baking soda. Drink 2 glasses of water. Then once every 20 minutes, drink another glass of water containing a teaspoon of baking soda. (The baking soda discourages bacterial growth and eases the stinging sensation). Relief should begin within 3 hours.

Relief of pain from painful bladder syndrome is also aided by the fact that baking soda increases the pH of urine.

Constipation
Old timers insist that drinking a glass of water mixed with a half teaspoon of baking soda is good for relieving

constipation.

Yeast Infections

To relieve the itching and burning of yeast infections, mix together 1 tablespoon baking soda in a glass of warm water and drink. Lemon juice can be added to flavor for taste, if necessary. Drink several glasses a day until infection is gone.

A warm baking soda soak can also help soothe the discomfort of yeast infections. Pour 1/2 cup of soda into warm bath water and soak for about 20 minutes two or three times per day until symptoms are relieved.

Loose Bowels

Try drinking a glass of water mixed with a half teaspoon of baking soda to regulate irregular bowels.

OUTSIDE THE BODY

Want to look younger and healthier without spending hundreds of dollars on the latest fad "star" treatment?

Would you like your skin to be petal-soft again without the high cost of heading off to the nearest salon?

Does nothing seem to work to rid yourself of that painful cold sore?

Do you struggle with body odor no matter how much you bath or shower?

Welcome to baking soda! Popular culture would have us believe we NEED expensive beauty products and lengthy regimens to make us beautiful. Simple soaps are being replaced by the latest 14-day "must have."

Spas are being opened on every corner touting the latest "technique" to bring back our youth.

Lunchtime facelifts are now commonplace, as our seaweed soaks and painted on "glows" to make us look our best.

And how many new beauty products crowd our shelves, but disappear after only a few months...once a newer and better version arrives? New and improved products are continually being introduced. Millions of dollars per year are spent convincing us we must have it! Billions of our hard earned dollars are being spent on keeping youthful. They tempt us with products to help every imperfection and condition under the sun.

Consider just a handful of the products we purchase on a regular basis. How many of these are worth the hype? How many products wind up in the bottom of a drawer, long forgotten about, never living up to the promise on the package?

- New and improved shampoos

- Must-have conditioners

- Luxurious baths and soaks

- The latest and greatest skin creams

- Expensive scrubs and lotions

- Perfumed powders and ointments

Who can keep up with it all?? And what about the latest "cures" on the market?

First, companies spend millions of dollars telling us why their product is the ONLY product that will cure whatever ails you. Only for them to come back, sometimes months later, spending millions more dollars trying to convince us the original product has now been "new and improved" and we must have it or we are missing out!

Enough is enough. It's time to get back to the simple basics of simple beauty! And the wonders of simple baking soda are simply wonderful!

Baking soda is a wonderful companion to the human body. It is 100% natural, and always soothing to the skin. It is non-irritating to sensitive skin and is a wholesome, chemical-free way to deodorize and freshen the body. It is gentle enough to use on our bodies every day without worrying about chemical buildup or residue or drying out our skin.

And, baking soda has long been used to treat everyday ailments, aches and pains. Baking soda's history goes back to long before health product and pharmaceutical companies picked up on its usefulness! They are doing what we have long known.

Baking soda is a natural remedy for so much of what troubles our bodies.

- Body and foot odor

- Burns

- Rashes

- Stings and Bites

- Athlete's Foot

- Nail fungus

- Dry, itchy skin

- Flaky scalp

No need to buy into whatever new miracle product manufacturers are selling this week. No need to immerse ourselves in expensive products or unpronounceable chemical compounds. We already know how amazing the simplicity of baking soda can be.

Soaks and Baths

A lukewarm bath with a half cup of baking soda added to it will help to soothe dry skin.

Add a handful of baking soda to bathwater to make your skin soft and youthful again.

A baking soda bath can help lessen skin irritations.

Make Your Own Bath Salts

Make your own bath salts. Mix 1 cup Epsom® salts, 1/3 cup baking soda, 2 cups coarse sea salt. Mix everything well and store in an airtight container. Several drops of perfume or a teaspoon of essential oil can be added for a relaxing, luxurious aroma.

Relieve Itchy Skin

Add a cup of baking soda to your bath water to make your skin smooth, silky and relieve itchy skin.

Renew dull skin by rubbing it with a paste of baking soda and water. Old skin will give way to healthy new cells.

Facial Compress

Make a baking soda facial cream by combining 2 parts baking soda to 1 part water. Rub in a gentle, circular motion around face and let set for five minutes. Rinse clean with warm water.

Pimples

Help keep pimples, blackheads and whiteheads away by using an occasional facial scrub. Gently rub baking soda paste using circles into your forehead, cheeks and chin. Rinse with warm water and pat dry. This exfoliation will help keep pimples and blackheads from forming.

Prickly Heat and Heat Rash

Use baking soda to relieve prickly heat and to prevent heat rash.

Soothe a Sunburn

Soak away the pain of sunburn by dissolving 1/2 cup baking soda into a tub of tepid water. Soak in this cool bath to relieve sunburn pain as often as it feels good!

Windburns

Summer windburns can be relieved by holding a cool baking soda compress against damaged and irritated skin.

Razor or Shaving Burns

Take the sting out of razor or shaving burns quickly and easily. Dissolve some baking soda in a dish of cool water. Dip a towel or a few cotton balls in the cool solution and gently wipe over irritated area of the skin.

Earwax

To remove earwax, flush the ear canal with this solution. Mix 1/4 teaspoon of baking soda with 2 tablespoons of warm (not hot) water. Pour into affected ear and allow to stay in ear 30 – 60 minutes. Baking soda solution will dissolve stubborn ear wax buildup.

To eliminate difficult earwax buildup, irrigate the ear canal with a solution combination of vinegar and baking soda to break up wax.

Pretty Powder
Fill a pretty container full of baking soda and add a few drops of your favorite perfume. Apply with a powder puff anytime you want to "freshen up"!

Elbows and Feet
Soften elbows and rough feet with a paste of baking soda and water or vinegar.

Foot Scrub
Use a baking soda scrub paste to remove dead skin from feet. Make a scrub paste by mixing baking soda and a little water. Pat dry with a soft towel. Can also be used on other problem areas, such as dry elbows.

Scour and clean children's ankles of the dirt that seems to cling even after bath time!

Footbaths
Give yourself a luxurious footbath by dissolving 1/2 cup of baking soda in a small pan of warm water. Soak your feet for 5 – 10 minutes.

Instead of purchasing expensive, and sometimes greasy, additives for your motorized footbath and massager, try this. Just add a handful of baking soda into the warm footbath water. The soft bubbling action in combination with baking soda will help keep your feet happy and healthy.

Foot Odor

To relieve foot odor, soak in a baking soda footbath at least twice a week. Adding a tea bag will produce a stronger, more effective soak.

Smelly shoes can be renewed by dusting the insides with baking soda and allowing them to rest overnight.

For tennis shoes and sneakers that trap odors easily, make a baking soda sachet and place in shoes between uses.

Athlete's Foot

To combat the itching of athlete's foot, dust your feet with baking soda. Don't forget to sprinkle baking soda inside your socks and shoes, as well.

For tougher cases of athlete's foot, make a baking soda cream using 1 tablespoon of baking soda and 1 – 2 teaspoons of water. Gently massage affected area between toes and let stand for 10 minutes. Rinse off and dry feet thoroughly. Dust shoes and socks before putting them on your feet.

Toenail Fungus

Toenail fungus can be cured by gently rubbing infected nails with a baking soda paste. Leave on for a few minutes and rinse clean with warm water. Dry well. Do this daily until fungus disappears. Also works with fungus on fingernails.

Relieve Tired, Itchy Skin

Smooth a light puff of baking soda over your body to ease itchy, dry skin.

Exfoliate

Want younger, more youthful skin? Remove old

cells by exfoliating once a week with this natural cream. Combine three parts baking soda to one part water and mix thoroughly. Cleanse face in a gentle, circular motion. Rinse in warm water and pat dry.

Add slightly more baking soda for a microdermabrasion treatment. Rinse in cool water and follow up with a moisturizer for youth-like results.

Cold and Mouth Sores

To eliminate painful and unsightly cold sores, apply a thick paste made of baking soda and water on the cold sore 2 – 3 times per day.

Rinse three times a day with warm water and baking soda to cure mouth sores.

Stains and Odors on Hands

Wet hands and rub together with baking soda to remove stains from hands. Works great on ground in dirt, too.

Does cooking leave your hands smelling like onions or garlic? Remove odors from hands by washing with a tablespoon or two of baking soda. This will also help leave your hands soft to the touch!

Keep Fingernails Beautiful

Help keep fingernails beautiful with a weekly massaging with baking soda paste. Using a circular motion, gently rub paste into nails, cuticle and nail bed. This will keep nails from discoloring and keep the nail bed healthy for good growth.

Body Odor

For body odor, dust with baking soda. You can also add crushed, dried basil leaves for a stronger deodorant.

Baking soda can be used as an odor-killing underarm wash.

Deodorant
Substitute baking soda for your store bought deodorant by applying it with a powder puff beneath your arms.

To make your own, personal deodorant, pour 1/4 cup of baking soda into a small canister. Add your favorite scented talc or a few drops of perfume. Apply daily with a powder puff, or as needed.

Exfoliate
Use baking soda as a gentle exfoliate for face and body. Works wonders on feet, too!

Sunburn
Dust baking soda on sunburn for instant relief and to soothe skin.

For painful sunburns, soak a clean cloth in a bowl of cold or icy water with 1/4 cup of baking soda. Place cool cloth over sunburned area.

Rash Relief
Relieve the irritation of rashes by bathing in warm water and a cup of baking soda.

Poison Ivy and Poison Sumac
Ease itching associated with poison ivy and sumac by soaking in a baking soda bath.

Stings and Bites
Baking soda paste can neutralize the venom of a wasp sting.

A homemade paste made of baking soda, just moistened with a touch of water, will take the ouch! out of a bee sting. First, gently remove stinger with a fingernail or a pair of tweezers. Cover the area with a thick coating of cool baking soda paste. Repeat whenever relief is needed.

Make Your Own Calamine Lotion

Combine 4 tablespoons baking soda with 2 tablespoons water and mix together in a small container. Apply this soothing cream to bug bites or sunburn for instant relief.

Oily Hair

For troublesome, oily hair, lightly sprinkle baking soda on a brush and run it through your hair. Blow excess away with a hair dryer.

Make Your Own Shampoo

Begin by mixing 1 tablespoon of baking soda 1 teaspoon of water. Add 1 tablespoon of lemon juice and a few drops of glycerine. Massage into scalp and rinse through hair. Rinse with fresh water a little apple cider vinegar.

Hair Detox

Use baking soda as a detox for hair product buildup. To remove buildup from using hair sprays and gels, once a month add a teaspoon or two of baking soda to your normal shampoo. Wash and rinse like normal.

Remove Buildup on Brushes and Combs

Residue on brushes and combs can be easily cleaned by soaking in a sink bath of warm water and baking soda.

Swimming Hair

After swimming in a chlorinated pool, revive hair with a baking soda rinse.

Dandruff

For dandruff, try baking soda instead of your normal shampoo. After wetting your hair, rub baking soda into your scalp, rinse, dry and style as usual. After several "washings" you should see a marked improvement in your scalp and along with softer, shiny hair.

Burns

For minor burns, pour baking soda into a bowl of cold or icy water. Soak a small cloth in the bowl and hold it on the burn area. As the cloth warms to your body temperature, repeat the process to keep it cold until the burning sensation ends. For added relief, add a tea bag to the water or use a cup or two of cooled tea to replace the water.

Diaper Rash

Help relieve diaper rash by adding a few tablespoons of baking soda to your baby's warm bathwater.

Cradle Cap and Itchy Scalp

Cradle cap or itchy, flaky scalp can be relieved by applying a soft cream made of 1 tablespoon of baking soda and 1 -2 teaspoons of water. Massage into baby's scalp and leave on several hours or overnight. Rinse clean. This safe treatment works equally well for babies, children and adults.

Wet a soft cloth and dip in baking soda to gently remove isolated spots of cradle cap.

Reduce a Baby's Fever

Baby have a fever? Help bring her fever down by bathing her in a tub of lukewarm water with a handful of baking soda added to it.

Eyebrows

Dip brow brush into baking soda and brush through brows for thicker, healthier, separated eyebrows. This is also a good way to remove all traces of cream foundations.

Jellyfish Sting

Use baking soda to help ooze out the venom of a painful jellyfish sting.

SOME IN MEDICAL SCIENCE SAY...

Sodium bicarbonate has been used for decades in the treatment of illness by the medical community. Research is continually being done to find new uses for this mineral --- on common and not-so-common illnesses. Because sodium bicarbonate has the ability to regulate pH levels in humans, it has opened the door to many potential new uses. Research studies continue to find more and more uses for this wondrous white mineral.

Because sodium bicarbonate (baking soda) naturally contains a high level of sodium, people with high blood pressure or who are on a salt restricted diet should avoid baking soda. At a minimum, consult your health care practitioner before beginning any use of baking soda a home remedy.

Kidney Disease

Chronic kidney disease may be slowed by the daily ingestion of baking soda. Studies have shown that since many kidney disease patients show a low level of bicarbonate in their system, a condition called metabolic acidosis, baking soda can help regulate that level and slow the disease's progression. Patients were given a daily tablet of sodium bicarbonate and showed that chronic kidney disease's progression was slowed by the addition. But, the tablet had to be given on a daily basis in order to be effective.

Cancer Sores

Often times when a patient suffering from cancer receives life-saving radiation treatment or chemotherapy, sores appear in the mouth as a result. These sores can be quite painful and relief can be difficult to find in the healing process.

Mouth sores caused from radiation treatment or chemotherapy can be eased by rinsing in a simple solution of salt, water and baking soda.

Simply make a baking soda rinse by mixing a small glass of warm water with 1 teaspoon of baking soda and a pinch of salt. Rinse around mouth and sore areas and spit out.

Any sores occurring on the outside of the mouth can be eased with a baking soda paste made of 1 tablespoon of baking soda and a teaspoon of water. Mix together and place over sore.

Blepharitis is a condition where the eyelash follicles along the eyelids become inflamed due to infection. Usually, the cause for this is that some of the bacteria that is normally found on the skin gets into the follicle itself. This presents itself as red, swollen, itchy eyelids. You can even find "dandruff" or flaky skin on the eyelashes themselves.

Soothe and disinfect swollen and blepharitis irritated eyelids with a compress soaked in water and baking soda for fast relief.

Take a clean, soft cloth and soak it in cool water and baking soda. Hold on the swollen eye area as often as needed. This will not only bring relief to the itchy swollen area, but the baking soda will act to combat the bacteria itself.

Conjunctivitis (Pink Eye)
Conjunctivitis, or pink eye, is reddening of the eye and is caused be either bacterial or viral infections. An itching sensation along with mucus discharge is associated with pink eye.

Because pink eye is highly contagious, and due to the fact we are dealing with such a sensitive area of the body as the eye, great care should be taken in dealing with pink eye.

Be sure every item that comes into contact with your eye, either directly or indirectly, is sterilized prior to using. This includes boiling and sterilizing the water you will be using as your solution base, measuring utensils and dropper or rinsing cup.

Mix 1/4 teaspoon of baking soda into 1/2 cup of sterilized water. Stir until baking soda is completely dissolved. With either a dropper or small rinsing up, use solution as a soothing eyewash and to kill offending bacteria. Gently pat eye area and face dry with a soft cloth after rinsing, and immediately wash cloths that have come into contact with eye area.

Tumors
Scientists are also studying the effect sodium bicarbonate may have on reducing the size of tumors in cancer patients.

The theory is that sodium, as we know, raises the

body's pH level and alkalinity. Since we know this raised alkaline environment is paramount in killing cancer cells, research is being done by injecting sodium bicarbonate directly into tumors and measuring their growth through MRIs and CT scans.

Asthma

Asthma is a chronic respiratory disorder in which the patient's airway becomes inflamed and narrows, making breathing difficult.

Asthma can be a life-threatening, debilitating disease in some of its youngest and most helpless patients. To make matters worse, some of these young patients find their asthma resistant to two of the most common modes of treatment, Corticosteroids and bronchodilators.

New research is regarding sodium bicarbonate is showing great promise as an alternative treatment for young asthmatic children when it is administered intravenously. Data indicates the intravenous form of baking soda can greatly improve lung function in children suffering from what can be a life-threatening illness. The addition of sodium bicarbonate can reduce respiratory distress and lowers excessive acidity in body fluids... ultimately making it easier to breathe.

Dehydration

Dehydration is the body's loss of water and necessary minerals for life. Dehydration can be a life-threatening condition brought on rapidly by a host of different circumstances:

- Diarrhea

- Sun exposure

- Burns

- Vomiting

- Overheating

Burn victims, as well as people suffering from dehydration can quickly find themselves in need of fluid replacement. Electrolyte replacement drinks, such as ones you would find on your grocer's store shelves, can be one way of replacing fluids and electrolytes quickly. Some have found that these "sports" drinks contain too much sugar and fall short of what is necessary to replace lost fluids in our bodies. Or, you may not have one of these drinks on hand at the time of emergency.

BUT, you do have the solution in your home pantry. Electrolyte and fluid replacement can be easily and quickly remedied at home with a few things from your pantry.

Mix one teaspoon of salt, 1/3 teaspoon of baking soda, 1 scant 1/4 cup of sugar and a quart of water. Shake in a bottle or stir in a pitcher. You can add flavorings, like lemon, if you choose.

Remember, once your body feels thirsty, it is already short on fluids. Always keep these simple, staple ingredients in your home in the case of an emergency.

Enhanced Performance or Risky Business?
Athletes have found a use for sodium bicarbonate in the world of athletic performance. Familiar to some as bicarbonate "doping" or as "buffering," baking soda is being used to boost performance in cyclists, runners and weight lifters.

The idea behind bicarbonate doping is that as

we exercise our muscles begin to produce a chemical compound known as lactic acid. As lactic acid builds, our muscles become fatigued. Athletes believe that by ingesting sodium bicarbonate, this mineral buffers acid in the muscles, allowing them to continue performing instead of becoming fatigued.

Due to some of the side effects associated with this type of athletic performance enhancement, such as bloating and fluid retention, most "true" athletes believe the temporary advantage received by bicarbonate doping is greatly offset and actually hinders performance. It is also believed that bicarbonate doping can cause vomiting, cramping and even be dangerous for your heart! As a matter of health, bicarbonate doping should ALWAYS be avoided.

Chapter Six

THE INCREDIBLE, EDIBLE SODIUM BICARBONATE: COOKING WITH SODA

BAKING SODA IS FOR BAKING

Modern baking soda's association with cooking dates back to the 1800s. 1835 saw the first successful baking powder compound with the addition of cream of tartar.

Since then, a host of other uses for baking soda in the kitchen have been developed. From baking delicious leavened breads to tenderizing that special cut of meat, making a crisp, thin texture known as tempura batter, or adding something extra to that special fizzy drink ...baking soda does it all. And in this chapter, you will find wonderful recipes for each of those...and more!

But first, a quick lesson in why baking soda does what it does so well!

How Does Baking Soda Work?

As you know, baking soda, or sodium bicarbonate, is a white alkali found in nature. Ancient Egyptians first mined and used this mineral as a soap. Through the ages, more and more uses were found for this soda, and in the 1800s, bakers began using baking soda as a leavening agent in breads.

Bakers found baking soda worked by trapping carbon dioxide in other ingredients used for baking bread, causing it to rise. Baking soda, as it came in contact with an acidic ingredient, would begin to effervesce (fizz), trapping carbon dioxide and forming bubbles. It was as the fizzing continued and bubbles were formed that the mixture would begin to rise. And, voila! A new leavening agent was born!

Bakers soon began making baking soda a staple ingredient in every baked good imaginable from homemade breads to cakes and pastries. And, as you know, baking soda has continued its use as a leavening agent in baked goods even today.

One of the earliest cooking uses of baking soda was in the form of soda bread (look for a delicious recipe later in this chapter!). This Irish bread, like so many breads made with baking soda, is a quick-rise bread that eliminates the demand for large amounts of kneading action.

Baking Soda or Baking Powder?

Both baking soda and baking powder, like yeast, are considered leavening agents. Usually, the two agents are not used together in the same recipe, since they behave differently when in contact with other ingredients.

Baking soda is the pure form of the mineral, sodium bicarbonate. This natural alkali is processed into a fine white powder. It reacts by effervescing, or fizzing, with acids. This "fizzing" action causes carbon dioxide bubbles to develop, which in turn, stimulate the leavening action it is most known for.

In order for the fizzing and rising action to take place, baking soda must mix with some form of acid. Citrus fruits, vinegar, chocolate, maple syrup, brown sugar, honey and cocoa are some of the most popular. Other ingredients with less prominent acidity can also be used. A few of these include molasses, yogurt, buttermilk or even sour cream. Baking soda's leavening action begins as soon as the ingredients are mixed, so remember that the batter needs to be cooked immediately.

Baking powder, on the other hand, is derived from the same sodium bicarbonate that is baking soda, but with acid salt additives. The most popular additives in baking powder are tartaric acid (or cream of tartar), calcium acid phosphate, sodium aluminum sulfate and some addition of a agent to aid in drying such as cornstarch. Different additives give us the difference between single-acting and double-acting baking powder.

The chemical reaction of the baking powder reacting with an acid takes place in both single- and double-acting baking powders. However, in single-acting powders, the reaction takes place only one time. And usually this reaction occurs in the beginning stages of preparation, such as mixing the ingredients together. In the case of double-acting powder, this reaction takes place in the initial mixing stages, but also again in the actual baking stage.

Shelf Life

Baking powder, if stored in a clean, sealed container and kept dry, has a substantially shorter shelf life than baking soda, and is also more expensive. Baking powder usually remains fresh for about a year after opening the container, while baking soda, stored correctly, lasts indefinitely.

SUBSTITUTIONS

Inevitably, we begin mixing a delicious recipe only to find out we have run out of a necessary ingredient, like baking powder or yeast. What should you do if you find yourself out of baking powder? Can baking soda be safely substituted?

Baking Powder

Baking soda, because it is truer in form than it's cousin baking powder, is about four times as effective as baking powder. And, because baking soda and baking powder are two different products with two different uses, they cannot be directly interchanged in recipes. But, baking soda can be mixed with a few other simple kitchen ingredients to make your own baking powder in an emergency. To make your own baking powder, try one of these.

Combine 1/3 teaspoon baking soda with 1/2 teaspoon cream of tartar and 1/8 teaspoon salt to make about 1 teaspoon of single-acting baking powder.

If cream of tartar is not available, you can also substitute baking powder by using other acidic means. Try this replacement.

Simply replace each teaspoon of baking powder with 1/4 teaspoon of baking soda and replace 1/2 cup of the recipe's liquid with an equal amount of any acidic liquid, such as sour milk or citrus juice.

For instance, if your recipe calls for 1 teaspoon of baking powder, you can replace the powder with 1/4 teaspoon of baking soda. But then you MUST remember to replace another liquid from the recipe (such as milk or water) and exchange it for something acidic in its place (such as lemon juice).

Another substitution for baking powder can made if cream of tartar is unavailable. Vinegar can be used in the place of cream of tartar.

Dry Yeast

Baking soda can also be used to replace the rising action in yeast. Mix 1/2 teaspoon baking soda and 1/2 teaspoon powdered vitamin C to take the place of 1 teaspoon dry yeast. Unlike dry yeast, baking soda is fast acting, so you need to bake your bread immediately after mixing.

Eggs or Oil

In the middle of preparing a cake mix, only to find you are out of both eggs and oil? Just use diet soda pop, such as Sprite or Dr. Pepper, in its place!

Sugar

Run out of sugar while baking? Substitute 3/4 cup honey for each cup of granulated sugar in a recipe. Then reduce another liquid in the recipe by 1/4 cup and add 1/4 teaspoon baking soda. This will help neutralize the acid in the honey. Reduce the oven temperature by 25°. Substituting honey for sugar alters the flavor and tends to make baked good moister, chewier and darker. But remember, **NEVER** feed raw honey to babies less than one year old due to the risk of botulism. Instead, try this substitute.

You can also try this substitution recipe using maple syrup in place of granulated sugar. Replace 3/4 cup of maple syrup plus 1/4 teaspoon of baking soda for each cup of granulated sugar. Reduce another liquid in the recipe by 3 tablespoons.

Buttermilk

An easy substitution can be made for buttermilk. To replace 1 cup of buttermilk, use 1 cup of milk plus 2 teaspoons of baking powder and 1/2 teaspoon of baking soda.

Caustic Soda

Caustic soda, also called washing soda, is not the same as baking soda. It is a strong alkali, and about four times as strong as baking soda.

A FEW WORDS ABOUT...

Using Baking Soda and Powder Together

Baking soda is alkaline, and when mixed with acidic ingredients, its reaction causes bubbles of carbon dioxide to be released. It is this reaction, when trapped inside batter, that helps baked goods to rise.

Baking powder, on the other hand, contains baking soda plus other acidic salts meant to react when they get wet or heated.

Some recipes call for both baking soda and powder. These recipes use the soda to offset the extra acidity in batters from ingredients such as buttermilk or molasses.

Baking soda can't be omitted from these recipes without altering the flavor or making the baked goods tough.

Cocoa Powder

Recipes call for all different types of cocoa powder, from Dutch cocoa to dark cocoa. Most baked goods list plain old "cocoa" as the ingredient of choice, which is non-alkalized. This cocoa is more acidic than Dutch cocoa. Most of the time, different types of cocoa are interchangeable within recipes, with little or no difference noted. However, if the recipe also includes baking soda, it may need the acidic action of cocoa to complete the necessary chemical reaction.

And, cocoa powder can never be used as a direct substitute for cocoa. Cocoa is a bitter ingredient, while cocoa powder is sweetened and is used as a cocoa beverage mix.

Tofu Noodles

Tofu noodles, which also go by the name soy noodles, are chewy noodles often used in soups or stir fry dinners. Tofu noodles that are purchased from the supermarket dry should be reconstituted before cooking for best results. You can soak them in a little water and baking soda until they regain their soft, chewy texture. Rinse them off before cooking.

Hartzhorn (Triebsalz, hartshorn, salt of hartshorn)

Hartzhorn is a distant ancestor of today's baking powder. It was originally derived from the ground antlers of reindeer. It can still be found in some German or Scandinavian stores or markets, since it is still an ingredient in some baking recipes. It is sometimes called "baker's ammonia" which has no relation to normal, household ammonia.

To make a substitution for 1 teaspoon baker's ammonia, or hartzhorn, try mixing 1 teaspoon baking powder plus 1 teaspoon baking soda.

Leavening

Leavening can be any substance that produces bubbles in batter or dough causing a rising action.

Most breads use yeast as their leaving agent. This process ferments sugar, which will produce the rising action of carbon dioxide.

Baking soda and powder are also used to leaven quick-rise breads, muffins, cookies and cakes. If there is not enough acid in the batter, the recipe will also ask for baking powder. This will combine with the baking soda and one or more acidic salts. As the baking powder becomes moist or rises in temperature, the soda will react with salt and release gas bubbles, causing the batter to rise.

Gaseous bubbles can also be trapped in egg whites as they are beaten. This form of leavening can be used in baking sponge or angel food cakes.

TOO MUCH OF A GOOD THING

Be cautious of using more baking soda than is required in a recipe. Too much baking soda in a recipe can cause the chemical reaction to take place too fast and too early in the culinary process. This leads to cakes that rise beautifully, only to have them fall before the baking period is complete.

Over use of this wonderful product can also make an otherwise scrumptious recipe bitter tasting. In addition, too much baking soda can also bring a coarse, crumbly texture that has a soapy sort of taste.

SPECIAL SECRETS

Have you ever wondered how bakers get a perfect rise to their cakes? Or how restaurant chefs always seem to prepare a crisp, golden skin on meat? What about restaurant vegetables that are served bright green instead of faded and dull?

Cooks and bakers all have their share of culinary secrets. This next section will share the secrets of some of those experts with tips on how to bring out the best in all of your dishes!

Red Velvet Cake

Did you ever think of how luscious Red Velvet Cakes are made? The secret is a combination of baking soda and cocoa used together resulting in that beautiful deep red chocolate color the dessert is famous for! (Shhh.... there is also a recipe for Red Velvet Cake in the recipe section of this book!)

Tenderize Meat

Tenderize pork or chicken by rubbing it with baking soda. Let stand for 10 minutes and rinse off.

Have a tough cut of meat? Tenderize beef by rubbing with baking soda and allowing to rest in the refrigerator 4 – 6 hours. Rinse soda off and cook.

Wild Game

Venison will lose its gamey taste if 1/2 teaspoon of baking soda is added to the water in which it is cooked. This also works on quail, wild turkey, bear and antelope, too.

When canning venison or other game, add a quick pinch of soda to each jar to get rid of that gamey taste.

Gutting Game

Hate the odor when you are gutting a deer or other wild game? Try sprinkling some baking soda into the gutted belly to absorb those odors.

Rhubarb

For milder rhubarb, add a pinch of baking soda to cooking water.

Prawns

Soak prawns for a quarter of an hour in a cup of water with a dash of baking soda added to it. Rinse before cooking.

Vegetables

A pinch of baking soda in the cooking water will help tenderize vegetables so they will cook faster. This works wonderfully on cabbage, broccoli, peas, carrots and string beans.

Vegetables cooked in water mixed with baking soda retain that beautiful green hue, though baking soda can make them mushier, if not watched closely. It can also cause them to lose some of their vitamins. Vitamins A and C are especially at risk.

Keep Green Vegetables Green

A pinch of baking soda added to the water in which a green vegetable is boiled will keep it bright green and appetizing. Great on broccoli and Brussels sprouts.

Dried Beans

Baking soda is often used to soften soybeans before cooking. It is also useful with any dried beans or peas.

A little soda in the cooking water will reduce the gas formed when eating most kind of beans. Do not forget to add a little to baked beans, too.

Cleaning Fruits and Vegetables

Add 3 – 4 tablespoons of baking soda to a large bowl of cold water to wash fresh produce.

You can also add baking soda to a brush or scrubber when cleaning vegetables such as potatoes or carrots. Rinse after cleaning

Cauliflower

Add a few tablespoons of baking soda to cauliflower's cooking water to keep the vegetable white and appetizing.

Canning

For safer canning of high-acid vegetables, such as tomatoes, add a teaspoon of baking soda to each quart jar.

Tomatoes

For recipes containing tomatoes, like pasta sauces, reduce the acid taste by adding a pinch of baking soda.

Thanksgiving Turkey

Rub down your Thanksgiving Turkey with baking soda to give it a nice, crispy skin.

Crispy Pork Chops and Chicken

Next time you make pork chops or chicken, try rubbing a little baking soda on the outside of the meat prior to cooking. This will not only lock in moisture, but also give that wonderful, crispy skin we all crave!

Goose

When roasting a goose, dust it with baking soda to ensure a crispy skin and a moist interior.

Fish

Soak fish with a heavy smell for 30 – 60 minutes in 1 quart of cold water with 2 tablespoons of baking soda added. Rinse and pat fillets dry.

Peking Duck

For perfect Peking Duck, massage baking soda into the bird's skin. It will cook up crisp and crusty.

Chicken

When de-feathering a chicken, add baking soda to the water to make removing feathers easier. Also cleans and tenderizes the skin.

Water

Does your water have a bad taste? Try adding a teaspoon to a gallon jug of water and shaking it well for a fresh taste.

Lemonade

Try a pinch of baking soda to lemonade or ice tea to prevent clouding.

Sports Drinks

Make your own sports drink substitution by adding a pinch of baking soda and salt to a bottle of water. You can also add lemon or a little flavored drink mix for extra taste.

Omelets

For fluffy omelets, add 1/2 teaspoon of baking soda to the omelet batter.

Scrambled Eggs

Add a pinch of baking soda to your scrambled eggs for light, fluffy eggs.

Pasta Sauces

Don't forget to add a pinch of baking soda to your pasta sauces to reduce the acidity in the tomatoes for a fresher, more authentic sauce.

A Few Words of Caution

Baking soda is a form of sodium. So, if you are on a reduced or sodium restricted diet, use baking soda with caution.

Overuse of baking soda can dilute the effectiveness of some vitamins. Always consult your physician before beginning a baking soda regimen.

Chapter Seven

EMILY'S MINI COOKBOOK

RECIPES

We have learned a few secrets on how to add that extra something to our special dishes. But now, enough talk! Time to get started on some delicious recipes of our own using baking soda!

WARNING: Baking soda, baking powder and salt are all forms of sodium. If you are on a reduced, or sodium restricted diet, use baking soda with caution.

Irish Soda Bread

3 1/4 cups flour
1/4 cup baking powder
1 t. salt
1 t. baking soda
1/2 c. sugar
1 egg
1 T. butter, melted
1 1/2 c. buttermilk

In a large bowl, combine flour, baking powder, salt and baking soda. In a medium bowl, beat egg and then add melted butter and buttermilk. Add egg mixture to dry ingredients, stirring until completely incorporated. Pour mixture into a greased loaf pan.

Bake at 350° for 50 – 60 minutes, until top is golden brown. Remove from oven and let cool 10 minutes before removing from pan.

Emily's note: *For a more personalized Irish Soda Bread recipe, add your favorite fruits like dark or golden raisins, dates or currants.*

Make an extra loaf to freeze for a special surprise for friends.

Soda Powered Power Bars

4	c. whole wheat flour
1 1/2	t. baking powder
1 1/2	t. baking soda
1 1/2	t. cinnamon
1	t. cloves
1	t. nutmeg
1	t. ginger
2	c. brown sugar, packed
3/4	c. olive oil
2	eggs
1	c. raisins
1/2	c. walnuts, chopped

In a large mixing bowl, combine flour, baking powder, baking soda, cinnamon, cloves, nutmeg, ginger and brown sugar. In a smaller bowl, whisk eggs and add olive oil. Add egg mixture to bowl of dry ingredients and stir together. Add raisins and chopped walnuts.

Chill for at least 1 hour.

Divide mixture into 6 equal parts. Shape into slightly flattened rolls that are approximately 1/2 inch by 14 inches.

Bake rolls at 375º for 10 – 15 minutes. Cut into handy lengths and cool.

Soda Biscuits

2 c. flour
1 t. baking soda
1 T. cream of tartar
1 t. vanilla
1/2 t. salt
1/3 c. shortening
3/4 c. buttermilk

Mix flour, baking soda, cream of tartar and salt together in a mixing bowl. Cut in shortening with a pastry blender or forks. Add buttermilk and vanilla, and stir until batter reaches dough consistency.

Roll out to a 1" thickness. Cut with round biscuit cutters and place 2" apart on a cookie sheet. Bake at 350º for 12 – 15 minutes or until golden brown.

Preston County Buckwheat Cakes

1/2 cake yeast or 1 envelope dry yeast
1 t. salt
1 qt. + 2 c. lukewarm water, divided
3 c. buckwheat flour
1/2 t. baking soda
1/2 t. baking powder
2 t. sugar

Mix cake yeast or dry yeast and salt in one quart of lukewarm water and let stand 5 minutes. Add buckwheat flour and stir, making a stiff batter. Cover and let stand overnight.

Dissolve baking soda, baking powder and sugar in 1 cup hot water and stir into resting batter. When well mixed, add another cup of warm water (enough to make a thin batter) and bake cakes on a hot griddle.

Emily's note: Save at least 1 cup of the batter for a starter next time! Buckwheat cakes are better after the batter has aged a while. Keep it in the refrigerator for about a week. To use, add 2 cups room temperature water and 1/2 teaspoon salt and enough buckwheat flour to make a stiff batter again. Cover and let stand overnight. In the morning, begin anew by dissolving baking soda, powder, etc. as before.

Tempura Batter

1   egg, beaten
1   c. water, cold
1/4 t. baking soda
1/4 t. salt
1   t. sugar
1   c. flour

Mix baking soda, salt, sugar and flour in a small bowl. In a larger bowl, mix beaten egg and cold water (water must be cold). Add flour mixture to wet ingredients and mix until all ingredients are incorporated.

Emily's note: This batter MUST be used cold. After mixing, dip your favorite meats or vegetables in batter to deep fry, just as you would see at your favorite oriental restaurant! Works great on shrimp, chicken, beef, cauliflower, sweet peas any of your favorite vegetables!

Deep fry in hot oil, until a light golden brown, for a crispy texture. Pat dry on a paper towel.

Red Velvet Cake

2 1/2 cups flour
1 1/2 c sugar
  1/4 t. salt
1 1/2 t. baking soda
    1 T. vinegar
    1 t. vanilla
    2 eggs
    3 T. cocoa
  12 T. butter, unsalted
    1 c. whole milk or buttermilk

Beat butter and sugar together in a mixing bowl on medium speed for 1-2 minutes, until fluffy. Set aside. Mix flour, baking soda, cocoa and salt in a small bowl.

Slowly, add flour mixture to butter and sugar and mix on slow until fully incorporated. In a separate bowl, mix milk (or buttermilk), eggs, vanilla and vinegar. Add milk mixture to cake batter and combine completely.

Pour batter into 2 greased and floured 9" cake pans. Bake on middle oven rack at 350° for 20-30 minutes, until toothpick inserted into center of cake comes out clean. Cool 10 minutes in pans. Remove cake from pans and cool completely on wire racks.

Frost layers with cream cheese frosting, and refrigerate until ready to serve.

Emily's note: *Try my cream cheese frosting with Red Velvet Cake.*

Emily's Cream Cheese Frosting

1   stick butter (at room temperature)
1   pkg cream cheese (8 oz)
3   c. confectioner's sugar
1   t. vanilla
    Pinch of salt
    Vanilla bean

Beat butter in a mixing bowl until smooth and combine with cream cheese, confectioner's sugar, vanilla and salt. Cream all ingredients together until the perfect spreading consistency. Add a little milk for creamier results.

As an extra special touch on Red Velvet Cake, you can also add the scrapings of the inside of a vanilla bean for a deeper, richer flavor.

Anzac "Soldier" Biscuits

1   c. flour
1   c. sugar
1   c. coconut
1   c. rolled oats
3   T. hot water
1   stick of butter, melted
1   t. baking soda
1   T. maple syrup

In a mixing bowl, combine flour, sugar, coconut and rolled oats. Add melted butter and stir until incorporated. In a small bowl, dissolve baking soda in hot water until fully dissolved, and then add to flour and butter mixture.

Spoon rounded teaspoonfuls onto baking sheet and bake at 375° for 9-11 minutes. Cool on a cooling rack until finished cooling.

Lemon Poppy Seed Muffins

2	c. flour
3	T. poppy seeds
1/2	t. baking soda
1/2	t. salt
1	t. baking powder
3/4	c. sugar
1	stick butter, unsalted
2	eggs
1	T. lemon juice
1	t. vanilla
1	c. plain yogurt

In a bowl, combine flour, poppy seeds, baking soda, salt and baking powder. With an electric mixer, cream butter and sugar together until creamy. Add eggs. Add lemon juice, vanilla and yogurt until mixture is a soft, creamy consistency. With a wooden spoon, gradually add flour mixture until incorporated, but be careful to not overbeat. Batter will be lumpy.

Spoon batter into muffin cups lined with paper liners. Bake at 350° for about 20 minutes.

Pryanik

1 1/2 c. + 2T flour, divided
  1/2 c. honey + extra for brushing on tops of cookies
  1/4 c. butter (1 stick)
    2 T. baking soda
  1/4 t. cardamom
  1/4 t. ginger
  1/4 t. cinnamon
  1/4 t. allspice
  1/8 t. salt
    1 t. vanilla
  3/4 c. jam
  1/2 c. water
  1/2 c. sugar

Sugar Glaze: Bring water to a boil. Stir in sugar and mix together until sugar is completely dissolved. Remove from heat and set aside to cool.

Mix 1 1/2 cups of flour in a mixing bowl with baking soda, cardamom, ginger, cinnamon, allspice and salt. Set aside.

Heat honey and butter over low heat until butter is melted and mixture has a thin syrup consistency. Add vanilla and stir well. Add flour mixture to honey mixture and knead together until a soft dough forms. Form into a large ball and cover with plastic wrap. Place dough in refrigerator for 1 hour.

Sprinkle 2T flour on a flat surface and flour rolling pin. Roll dough to 1/8" thickness. Cut into rectangular shaped pieces using either a knife or fluted pastry wheel. Spread jam over one half of each rectangle. Fold dough in half over the jam and seal the edges together to lock in jam.

With a brush, "paint" cookie tops with a bit of honey for beautiful color and flavor.

Place cookies on a greased baking sheet and bake at 350° for 10-15 minutes. Remove from baking sheet and cool completely on wire rack. When cool, drizzle with sugar glaze.

Emily's note: Feel free to experiment with other spices such as cloves or even cayenne pepper for a little punch. You can also top these with your favorite chopped nuts or berries to personalize your own recipe! Some people even use a confectioner's sugar frosting drizzled over the tops!

Raisin Soda Bread

- 4 c. flour
- 2 T. sugar
- 1 t. baking soda
- 1 t. salt
- 1 t. cream of tartar
- 1 c. seedless raisins
- 1 1/4 c. buttermilk (or whole milk)
  Orange juice

Mix flour, sugar, baking soda, salt and cream of tartar in a large bowl. Stir in raisins and buttermilk. Knead on a very lightly floured surface into a soft, flat ball.

Cut a crisscross design in the top of the bread dough and bake in an oven at 400° for 20-30 minutes.

Wrap in a towel dampened with orange juice and allow the bread to cool before cutting.

Emily's note: You can brush on a little extra buttermilk on the top of the loaf prior to baking, if you wish.

Crepes

2 1/3 c. milk
1 1/2 c. flour
   3 eggs, slightly beaten
   2 T. sugar
   1 T. baking soda
   1 T. vinegar
 1/2 t. salt
   1 T. melted butter
     Olive oil

Combine baking soda and vinegar in a small bowl. Set aside. In a mixing bowl, stir together milk, flour, eggs, sugar and melted butter. Add in baking soda mixture. Place in refrigerator for one hour.

Heat pan coated in olive oil until very hot. Pour a small amount of batter into the pan and swirl to coat the bottom of pan. Cook 30 – 40 seconds and then gently flip over. Cook the second side 10 – 15 seconds, until set. Allow to cool separately so crepes do not stick together.

Once cooled, fill with your favorite filling!

Emily's note: *These crepes are delicious filled with creamed chicken as a special dinner entrée, or strawberry sauce served with real whipped cream for a luscious summer dessert!*

World's Best Caramel Corn

2	c. brown sugar
1/2	c Karo syrup (either light or dark)
1/2	t. cream of tartar
1/2	t. salt
1	c. butter or margarine (2 sticks)
1	t. baking soda
8-10	quarts unsalted popcorn (popped)

In a large pot, bring to a boil brown sugar, Karo syrup, cream of tartar, salt and butter or margarine. Continue boiling 3 minutes. Stir in the baking soda. As the soda begins to work, it will foam up in your pot. After mixture foams, turn off the heat, add popcorn and mix together. Pour out onto baking sheets and bake at 200° for 1 1/2 hours, stirring every 15 minutes. Take out of oven and cool, storing this sweet treat in a dry, covered container.

Emily's note: *As a special bonus, try adding peanuts or your favorite other nuts in with the popcorn mixture prior to baking!*

Soft Pretzels

1 1/4 c. warm water
   1 pkg. dry, active yeast
   1 t. sugar
  1/2 c. sugar
4 1/2 c. flour
1 1/2 t. kosher salt
   1 T. vegetable oil

Topping
1/2 c. baking soda
  4 c. hot water
1/4 c. kosher salt

In a small bowl, pour warm water heated to about 110°. Dissolve yeast and sugar into warm water and let stand 10 minutes.

In a large bowl, mix flour, sugar and salt. Make a small well in the center of dry ingredients and add oil and yeast mixture. Knead into a ball. If ball is too dry, add more water, one teaspoon at a time. Knead until smooth, about 8 – 10 minutes.

Coat the inside of a bowl with vegetable oil and place kneaded dough in it. Cover with a dish towel and place in a warm place. Allow the dough to rise to double its original size. This should take about an hour.

Mix baking soda in hot water. Carefully roll out dough into long "snakes" keeping them at least an inch thick. Form into large pretzel shapes and dip each one into the hot water and baking soda mixture. Place on a baking sheet and sprinkle heavily with kosher or sea salt.

Bake in hot oven at 425° for 8 - 10 minutes until golden brown.

Emily's note: *You can substitute pretzel salt for kosher salt in the topping. Pretzel salt has slightly larger crystals and is coarser than either kosher or sea salt.*

Texas Sheet Cake

```
    1  c. butter or margarine
    4  T. cocoa
    1  c. water
    2  c. flour
    2  c. sugar
  1/2  c. buttermilk or sour milk
    1  t. baking soda
1 1/2  t. cinnamon
    2  t. vanilla
    2  eggs
```

In a mixing bowl, combine flour, sugar, buttermilk, baking soda, cinnamon, vanilla and eggs.

Using a small saucepan, boil together, water, cocoa and butter or margarine. Pour water mixture into dry ingredients and mix thoroughly. Pour batter into a lightly greased and floured jelly roll pan.

Bake at 350° for 20 minutes, until center of cake springs back when touched. Move jelly roll pan to a wire rack until completely cool.

Emily's note: *Prepare this delicious frosting to use with your Texas sheet cake. A cookie sheet with turned up edges also works well for baking this yummy cake.*

Chocolate-Cinnamon Frosting

1/2 cup butter (1 stick), softened
1/3 c. milk
  3 c. confectioner's sugar
1/4 c. cocoa
  2 t. vanilla
1/2 t. cinnamon
1/2 c. chopped pecans, toasted

In a mixing bowl, cream butter and sugar together. Add in cocoa, cinnamon and vanilla. Slowly pour in milk and blend.

Frost cake and sprinkle with pecans.

Emily's note: *Don't worry if you are not a fan of pecans. This wonderful frosting is just as good without the nuts!*

Chapter Eight

BAKING SODA BEVERAGES

BEVERAGES

The idea of using baking soda in beverages is nothing new. In fact, that is just one of the ways soda shops of old gave their beverages that wonderful, fizzy taste.

There are many names beverages are known by which use the concept of "fizzy" drinks. Club soda, soda water, carbonated water, sparkling seltzer, sparkling water are all made by adding a small amount of baking soda to the water and then "charging" it with carbon dioxide. As the carbon dioxide begins to react, bubbles are created and voila...the fizzy drinks we love!

A Step Back in Time

Sometimes called effervescent soda, those old fashioned fountain sodas used soda bicarbonate as the final touch on their fountain drinks. Because the fizz didn't last long, customers needed to drink their sodas immediately to enjoy the effect. You can duplicate some of those old-fashioned and almost-forgotten recipes right here! Plus, you will find a new twist on a few old recipes just to keep things fun!

Just as in baking with soda, beverages use

the same effervescent reaction to pull off that fizzy action. The baking soda added to a beverage must have an acid to work with. Together, the two ingredients produce fizz and froth to make beverages something special.

A few things to remember:

- Most of these drinks work best if the water or base liquid is very cold. You'll find the drinks are more refreshing that way!

- The effervescent reaction once baking soda is mixed into your acidic beverage does not last long. So, make sure baking soda is the last ingredient added, just before serving.

- Do not try to add extra baking soda to make greater fizz or repeat the fizzing action. There is just enough soda in the recipes to create fizz, but adding more may make your beverages taste bitter.

- Because fizzy sodas derive their fizz from baking soda and not true fermentation, these beverages contain no alcohol. So, they are safe for children to enjoy!

- Remember that just like in cooking, baking soda used in beverages will need some sort of acid to react with. A few great ones in drinks include lemon juice, orange juice, sugar, cocoa or chocolate sauce, molasses and honey. After trying a few of these, why not try making up your own?

So, pull up a stool at the counter and take a step back in time with a few wonderful fizzy drinks... compliments of baking soda!

Word to the wise: do not use these or other carbonated beverages just before a singing performance. They will put air in your stomach and could lead to some very embarrassing public burping!

Fizzy Lemonade

1/4 cup lemon juice
1/4 cup cold water
2 T. sugar
1 t. baking soda

Combine lemon juice, water and sugar in a glass. Stir in baking soda.

Lemon-Grenadine Fizz

1/4 cup lemon juice
1/4 cup cold water
1 T. sugar
1 1/2 t. grenadine syrup
Crushed ice cubes
1 t. baking soda

Fill a drinking glass half full of crushed ice cubes. Pour lemon juice, water and sugar over the ice. Add grenadine. Stir in baking soda and enjoy!

Cherry Lemonade

1 cup lemon-lime soda, cold
2 T. cherry juice
1/4 c. lemon juice
1 T. sugar
Ice cubes
1 1/2 t. baking soda
1 maraschino cherry

Combine soda, cherry and lemon juice, and sugar in a tall glass with a few ice cubes. Add baking soda and stir. Use a maraschino cherry on top for eye appeal!

Old Fashioned Cream Soda

```
    1  can club soda, cold
  1/4  c. half and half
  1/4  c. chocolate syrup
    1  t. brown sugar
1 1/2  t. baking soda
       Real whipped cream
    1  maraschino cherry
```

In a tall glass, mix club soda, half and half, chocolate syrup and brown sugar. When combined, stir in the baking soda. Top with whipped cream and a maraschino cherry. Serve immediately!

Emily's note: Love the taste of old fashioned ice cream sodas? Just add a scoop of your best vanilla ice cream to this drink before topping with whipped cream and a cherry for a refreshing summertime dessert!

Orange Cherry Soda Fizz

```
    1  c. orange juice, cold
  1/4  c. lemon juice
  1/4  c. cherry juice (from a maraschino cherry jar)
    1  T. sugar
1 1/2  t. baking soda
    3  maraschino cherries
```

Mix orange, lemon and cherry juices in a large glass. Add sugar, baking soda and cherries. Serve immediately.

Tropical Fizz

1/2 c. orange juice
1/2 c. pineapple juice
 3   T. lemon juice
 1   T. sugar
1 1/2 t. baking soda
     Crushed ice cubes
 3   maraschino cherries

Fill a tall glass half full of crushed ice. Combine orange, pineapple and lemon juices and pour over crushed ice. Add sugar. Stir in baking soda and cherries and serve immediately.

Honey Lemonade

1/4 c. honey
1/4 c. lemon juice
1/2 c. cold water
 1   t. baking soda

Mix honey, lemon juice and cold water in a glass. Add baking soda and enjoy.

Emily's note: This drink can actually be served warm. It makes a wonderful home remedy for a sore throat. Just substitute boiling water for cold water.

Electrolyte Replacement Sports Drink

This essential drink is not only perfect for competitive athletes, but also during illnesses where dehydration is a concern.

```
1    qt. water
1/2  t. baking soda
1/4  c. sugar
1    t. salt
```

Mix baking soda, sugar and salt into a quart of water. Shake in a bottle or stir in a pitcher. For added flavorings, add the juice of a lemon or your favorite powder of flavored drink mix.

OTHER USES FOR BAKING SODA IN BEVERAGES

Water
Water taste funny? Try adding a pinch of baking soda to rid your water of any unpleasant alkaline taste.

Ice Cubes
A small amount of baking soda can be added to ice cubes to prevent freezer odors from contaminating your ice cubes.

Coffee
Add a pinch of baking soda to brewed coffee to neutralize its acid and there will be no more stomach pain while drinking coffee.

Milk
To keep milk from spoiling so fast, put a pinch of baking soda in the carton.

Chapter Nine

SODA SCIENCE AND FIZZY FUN

So far, we have discovered some practical uses for baking soda, ranging from cooking and cleaning to beautifying and baking. Now it's time to roll up our sleeves and have some fun!

Baking soda's effervescent property that releases carbon dioxide gas makes it a perfect medium for children's fun.

All we need is a little baking soda, some kind of an acid and plenty of room to make a mess! And, a fun spirit is definitely a must! You may want to plan many of these activities as outdoor fun. A few things to keep in mind:

- Be sure of your surroundings. Keep a safe distance from others, windows and pets.

- Eye protection goggles are recommended.

- As with any science project, make sure there is adequate adult supervision.

- Read through all of the instructions before beginning your project. Some of the action happens very quickly and you will want to be ready.

- Most of all, have fun! Let your creativity soar as you come up with baking soda science activities of your own!

Stoichiometry Science!

This is a fun way to get children interested in science. The idea is to make a fizzy drink of your own, similar to those that would be store bought...all with a little baking soda, and a lot of science.

Supply list:

1   lemon
1   t. baking soda
1   T. sugar
    Cold water
    Drinking glass

In a drinking glass, squeeze all of the juice from the lemon. Pour in identical amount of water to match lemon juice. Stir in sugar. Add baking soda and stir. The fizzing action begins as soon as the baking soda hits the acidity of the lemon juice. Now give it a taste!

Why it Works

Baking soda is a mineral found in nature. When this wonderful mineral, which acts as a base, comes in contact with the lemon juice, an acid, it begins to effervesce, or form bubbles. These are carbon dioxide bubbles that simulate "fizz" found in carbonated drinks!

Test the Acidity of Vinegar

How strong is your homemade vinegar? Commercial vinegar's acid content is standardized, but homemade vinegars can vary. What follows is one way to determine the percent of acid in a batch of vinegar.

Supply List:
1/2 c. water
  2 t. baking soda
1/4 c. water from a head of cooked red cabbage
  2 drinking glasses
     White vinegar

Mix 1/2 cup of water and 2 teaspoons of baking soda together. Add in water from red cabbage. Put 1/2 cup of clear water into each of 2 clear glasses. Add 1/8 cup of cabbage water to each glass. Use a glass dropper to put 7 drops of white vinegar from the supermarket into one glass of the cabbage flavored water. Thoroughly rinse the dropper.

Put 20 drops of the soda water into the same glass and stir well with a plastic spoon (not metal). The water will turn blue.

Now mix 7 drops of your vinegar into the second glass of the cabbage flavored water. Thoroughly rinse this dropper.

Add baking soda water to your vinegar and cabbage water, 1 drop at a time. Stir after each drop. Count the drops. When the color of your vinegar water turns the same shade of blue as the commercial vinegar water, the acid content of the two glasses will match.

To find the percent of acid in your vinegar, divide the number of drops of soda water you added to it by four. For example, if you added 20 drops of soda water to your vinegar, divide by four and find that the acid content is 5%. (The same as most super market vinegars.) The more soda water it takes to make your vinegar match the color of the vinegar control, the stronger your vinegar is.

Creating Carbon Dioxide Gases

Can the simple substance, baking soda, really create a gas? Try this experiment to find out.

Supply List

    Plastic self-sealing bag
1/4 c. lemon juice
  1 t. baking soda

Pour lemon juice into a plastic bag that can be sealed shut. Dump in baking soda and quickly seal the bag. Gently swirl the bag to be sure all of the baking soda is coated in lemon juice. Set aside and watch as the plastic bag expands with the newly created carbon dioxide gas!

Exploding Cork Shooters

This is a fun experiment that demonstrates the rapid build up of carbon dioxide gas. But, remember this happens quick, so be sure and do the experiment in a safe place, and point the bottle AWAY from yourself and anyone else in the room!

Oh, and safety goggles are highly recommended!

Supply List

Plastic pop bottle OR glass wine bottle, emptied
Cork (to fit bottle)
1/3 c. lemon juice
 1 T. baking soda
Safety goggles

Make sure cork fits bottle opening. Pour the lemon juice into the bottle. Carefully dump the baking soda into the bottle with the lemon juice and quickly replace the cork. KEEP BOTTLE POINTING IN A SAFE DIRECTION...DO NOT HOLD BOTTLE NEAR YOUR FACE AS YOU ARE PUSHING THE CORK ON. Gently swirl bottle contents and watch cork blow!

Baking Soda Lowers Water Temps

This demonstrates how water temperatures can be lowered through the use of the mineral sodium bicarbonate, or baking soda.

Supply List

2 water glasses
1 T. baking soda
Pitcher of water
Thermometer (digital works best)

Pour equal amounts of water into two drinking glasses. Water should come from the same source, for example a pitcher, so water temperatures are consistent. Stir 1 tablespoon of baking soda into ONE of the glasses. Take temperature readings from both glasses.

Baking Soda Boats

This is a great activity to launch in a pond or stream...or even your bathtub!

Supply List

1   2-liter plastic bottle
2   T. Baking soda
    Vinegar
    Nail
    Small rocks or gravel (must be able to fit thru bottle)
    Toilet paper

Take your empty bottle and, using the nail, poke a hole in the cap. Lay the bottle on its side and add rocks or gravel. There should be enough weight to cause the bottle to tip, leaving the bottle neck and cap in the water.

Fill the bottle 1/4 full of vinegar. Next, take 4 sheets of toilet paper and fill them with baking soda. Fold the toilet paper in all directions to protect the soda. If you need to, you can divide the soda between two sets of sheets.

Place your bottle near the water, and have the cap ready. Do not allow water to enter bottle. Quickly put baking soda packet into the bottle and close with the cap. Rocks should be weighting the bottles cap into the water. Watch it go!!

Baking Soda Submarine

This is similar to the Baking Soda Boat, but uses more weight to hold it down.

Supply List

1 1-liter plastic bottle
2 T. Baking soda
   Vinegar
   Nail
   Small rocks or gravel (must be able to fit thru bottle)
   Toilet paper

Take your empty bottle and, using the nail, gently poke a hole in the cap. Lay bottle on its side and add rocks or gravel. Do not fill the bottle with rocks. There should be enough weight to cause the bottle to stay beneath water, but not enough that it can't move in the water.

Fill the bottle 1/4 full of vinegar. Next, take 4 sheets of toilet paper and fill with baking soda. Fold toilet paper in all directions to protect soda. If you need to, you can divide the soda between two sets of sheets.

Place your bottle near the water, and have the cap ready. Do not allow water to enter bottle. Quickly put baking soda packet into bottle and close with cap.

Watch it go!!

Floating Bubbles

This is a fun experiment for small children who love bubbles. Watch these bubbles fly in the air as the children blow on them!

Supply List

1/2 c. vinegar
  2 T. baking soda
    Clear drinking glass
    Water
    Liquid dish soap
    Straw

In a clear glass, put 1/2 c. vinegar. Add two tablespoons of baking soda and begin blowing into the mixture with a straw. Watch the bubbles begin to float into the air. Now, try adding a few drops of liquid soap added to it...continue blowing air through the straw!

Erupting Volcano

This is a great science experiment and craft all in one! It takes a bit of time and needs to be done in stages, so carve out a little time and have some fun with it!

Supply List

Volcano
6 c. flour
2 c. salt
2 c. water
4 T. vegetable oil
1 2-liter soda bottle, emptied
   Paint, if wanted

Lava (erupting portion of the craft)
  Liquid dish detergent
2 T. baking soda
  White vinegar
  Red food coloring
  Funnel

First, we'll make the volcano. Combine flour, salt, water and vegetable oil in a large bowl. Mix together until all ingredients are incorporated and mixture is smooth and firm, about the consistency of wet clay.

Stand the empty soda bottle upright, and begin molding the "clay" mixture around the bottle, forming a volcano shape. Leave the bottle opening uncovered and undisturbed, but the cone of the volcano should reach the top of the bottle. Be sure not to drop any of the clay mixture into the bottle. Feel free to sculpt your volcano with "ravines" and "bumps." If desired, you can even paint your volcano to make it look more realistic!

Carefully pour water with a few drops of red food coloring into volcano's bottle, filling it almost to the top. Add a few drops of dish detergent. Pour the baking soda into the bottle.

When you are ready to "erupt" your volcano, pour vinegar directly into the volcano's bottle...and watch out!

Baking Soda Balloons

Watch baking soda blow up a balloon using its effervescent "fizzing" action!

Supply List

    Empty bottle, either plastic or glass
1   balloon
4   T. vinegar
2   T. baking soda
    Funnel

Place the bottle on a level surface and pour in vinegar using a funnel, if necessary. Take a balloon and gently pour baking soda into the bottom of the balloon. Without allowing the baking soda to fall into the vinegar bottle, put balloon over the bottle's neck.

Now hold the balloon upright so the baking soda falls into the bottle and vinegar. Watch the balloon fill with carbon dioxide gas!

Baking Soda Rocket

This is great outdoor fun. Be sure and keep clear of windows or other breakables, and do not "fire" your rocket near people. Read over these directions completely before beginning your rocket. The launching action takes place rapidly!!

Supply List

1   bottle with a non-screw cap or cork, empty
1   straw
    Vinegar
2   T. baking soda
    Plastic wrap
    Stick or wire, needs to fit inside straw

Place thin stick or wire in ground, a safe distance from houses, windows, cars or people. Tape straw to outside of bottle making sure straw is level with top of bottle. Pour 1" vinegar in bottle. Gently pour baking soda into a small square of baking soda.

When ready to launch, gently wad up plastic with soda (do not tie in knot....needs to open easily) and place in bottle. Put on cap or cork, but not too tight. Gently shake bottle to begin mixture. Turn bottle upside down and place straw over wire "launcher."

As baking soda and vinegar rapidly mix, carbon dioxide bubbles will be created and pressure will launch your rocket!

Baking Soda Bombs

Make sure you try this one outside...it makes a real mess!

Supply List

1 1/2 T. baking soda
      Plastic self-sealing bag
  1/2 c. Vinegar
      Paper towel

Cut a paper towel into a 4" x 4" square. Put baking soda in center of square and fold several times in all directions so soda is inside.

Pour vinegar into the plastic bag that you can seal shut. Carefully place the paper towel square in the bag, but do not allow it to touch the liquid...hold it with your fingers against the bag until the bag is closed and you are ready to launch your "bomb."

Let the baking soda towel drop into the vinegar solution and shake gently. The bag will rapidly expand and "pop!"

Sculpting Clay

Make batches of this clay to mold and have fun with on a rainy day.

Supply List

    2 c. baking soda
    1 c. corn starch
1 1/4 c. water
      Food coloring

Mix together baking soda and cornstarch in a pan. Add water and cook, stirring constantly, on medium heat 12-15 minutes. Mixture should be the consistency of mashed potatoes.

Remove from heat and allow to become cool to the touch. It's best to cover the clay with a damp rag so it won't dry out as it is cooling. Once clay is cool, you can separate it into different bowls and add the food coloring of your choice.

Baking soda clay can be made ahead and stored up to a week in your refrigerator. Just wrap it in plastic, or store in a sealed plastic bag. Remember to bring the clay back to room temperature by laying it out for an hour or two before using it.

Drying Your Clay Creations

There are several ways you can dry your finished creations. Simply air dry the clay by leaving it out overnight. For faster drying, preheat oven to 200º. Once heated, turn the oven off and place your clay creations inside for 10-15 minutes, depending on the size. Try not to over dry your clay pieces in the oven, as this may lead to cracking.

Once your creation is dry, you can decorate it with markers and paints, or add on beads with a hot glue gun.

Emily's note: *If you would like to put holes in your clay creation, remember to do it BEFORE drying your piece. Otherwise, it may crack or break when you try to pierce it.*

See the next page for fun ideas to create with your new clay!

Clay Creations
Wonderful treasurers you can make from your new baking soda clay!

After your ornament is dry, paint or color with brightly colored markers. Clear acrylic spray can be added to preserve and protect your new pieces. Add a beautiful ribbon to hang from a tree.

Christmas Tree Ornaments
Roll out your clay dough with a rolling pin to 1/4 inch thickness. Ornaments can be cut with a cookie cutter, or free form shaped with a knife. Be sure and put a hole in the ornament for a hanging ribbon before drying. Add a beautiful ribbon to hang from the Christmas tree.

Bead Jewelry
Clay beads can be formed by rolling clay into small balls of various shapes and sizes. To make a hole for stringing, carefully use a toothpick to poke holes through beads. Allow beads to dry fully before stringing together. You may want to knot string in between beads to protect them and keep beads from cracking against each other.

Photo Frame
Roll out clay dough to a 1/2 inch thickness. Cut out a rectangle from the dough. Cut out hole from frame slightly smaller than photo you wish to frame.

After drying and decorating, you can either glue a hook on the back for hanging, or use another piece of clay to make a stand.

Wall Letters
Roll out clay dough to a 1/2" thickness with a rolling pin. Use a knife to cut out large free form letters. After drying, paint letters and glue hooks to their backs for

hanging.

You can decorate a child's room with his name, or put a fun quote on the wall.

Child's Handprint
Roll out clay dough to a 1/2" thickness with a rolling pin. A freeform lump of clay can also be used. While clay is still wet, press child's hand into the clay.

Winter Village
Roll out clay dough to a 1/2" thickness with a rolling pin. Use a knife to cut out pieces to form houses resembling gingerbread houses.

After drying pieces completely, glue houses together. Paint and display with baking soda "snow" during the holiday season as your own Christmas village.

Clay Critters
Use fresh clay to form critter shapes and paint. Don't worry if a piece falls off as it is drying. Simply glue it back into place!

Napkin Rings
Roll out clay dough to a 1/4 inch thickness with a rolling pin. Use a knife to cut strips of clay into whatever width you want your napkin rings to be. Cut off desired length and roll into a ring. You may need to moisten the ends to completely seal the rings together. Place upright to dry,

Refrigerator Magnet
Refrigerator magnets can be made from any clay design. Just roll it out with a rolling pin and cut with a cookie cutter or knife to shape, or free form a shape to look like your favorite animal. Be sure you have given it

a flat "back." After your creation is completely dry, glue a magnet to the back.

Pins

Make a beautiful custom pin out of baking soda clay and paint. Glitter can be added into the wet paint, or put on with a glue wash when dry. Spray with acrylic coating to protect, and add a pin backing to the backside to complete.

Thank You!

No single book could contain all the fantastic uses, remedies or recipes, or fun that baking soda brings. I'm sure you have your own special recipe that depends on baking soda as its special, secret ingredient.

So, we would love to hear from you! If you have a natural remedy, cleaning and deodorizing method or scrumptious recipe you would like to share with others, please use this page to share it with me! If I use it in an upcoming edition of one of my books, I will send you a free copy of the new book upon printing.

If the form in this book isn't available, please feel free to just use a plain sheet of paper and mail it to us!

Thank you, and my best wishes for a long and healthy life.

Emily Thacker.

Emily, here is one of my favorite uses for baking soda:

_____
_____
_____
_____
_____
_____

❑ Yes, please credit this remedy to

_____
_____

❑ No, please use my remedy, but do not use my name in
the book. Either way, yes or no, if I use your remedy.
I'll send you a free copy of the new edition of home
remedies.

Your remedy can be one which uses baking soda or
simply one that you feel others would like to know about.

My favorite chapter in "The Baking Soda Book" is:

_____
_____

The most helpful remedy I appreciated in "The
Baking Soda Book" is

_____
_____
_____
_____
_____
_____

What I liked best about "The Baking Soda Book" is

_____
_____
_____
_____
_____
_____
_____

Would you be interested in hearing about my new
cookbook when it becomes available?

_____

My name and mailing address is:

_____
_____
_____
_____

If you have any comments or experiences to add
to the information you've read in this collection, or if you
have information for subsequent editions, please address
your letters to:

Emily Thacker
PO Box 980
Hartville, OH 44632

✂ please cut here

The Magic of Baking Soda

The Magic

of

Baking Soda

By Emily Thacker

90-DAY MONEY-BACK GUARANTEE

☐ **YES!** Please rush _____ additional copies of The Magic of Baking Soda and my FREE copy of the bonus booklet "72 Secrets To Look Younger" for only $12.95 plus $3.98 postage & handling. I understand that I must be completely satisfied or I can return it within 90 days for a full and prompt refund of my purchase price. The FREE gift is mine to keep regardless. *Want to save even more?* Do a favor for a close relative or friend and order two books for only $20 postpaid.

I am enclosing $ _____ by: ☐ Check ☐ Money Order (Make checks payable to James Direct, Inc.)

Charge my credit card Signature _____

[VISA] [MasterCard] [Discover] [AMEX]

Card No. _____ Exp. date _____

Name _____

Address _____

City _____ State _____ Zip _____

Mail To: JAMES DIRECT, INC. • PO Box 980, Dept. BA124 Hartville, Ohio 44632 • http://www.jamesdirect.com

✂ please cut here

Use this coupon to order "The Magic of Baking Soda" for a friend or family member -- or copy the ordering information onto a plain piece of paper and mail to:

The Magic of Baking Soda
Dept. BA124
PO Box 980
Hartville, Ohio 44632

Preferred Customer Reorder Form

Order this...	If you want a book on...	Cost...	Number of Copies...
The Magic of Baking Soda	*Plain Old Baking Soda A Drugstore in A Box?* Doctors & researchers have discovered baking soda has amazing healing properties! Over 600 health & Household Hints. *Great Recipes Too!*	$9.95	
The Vinegar Anniversary Book	Completely updated with the latest research and brand new remedies and uses for apple cider vinegar. Handsome coffee table collector's edition you'll be proud to display.	$9.95	
Amish Gardening Secrets	You too can learn the special gardening secrets the Amish use to produce huge tomato plants and bountiful harvests. Information packed 800-plus collection for you to tinker with and enjoy.	$9.95	
The Magic of Hydrogen Peroxide	An Ounce of Hydrogen Peroxide is worth a Pound of Cure! Hundreds of health cures, household uses & home remedy uses for hydrogen peroxide contained in this breakthrough volume.	$9.95	
The Vinegar Home Guide	Learn how to clean and freshen with natural, environmentally-safe vinegar in the house, garden and laundry. Plus, delicious home-style recipes!	$9.95	

Any combination of the above $9.95 items qualifies for the following discounts...

	Total NUMBER of $9.95 items	

Order any 2 items for: $15.95

Order any 3 items for: $19.95

Order any 4 items for: $24.95

Order any 5 items for: $29.95

Order any 6 items for: $34.95 and receive 7th item FREE

Any additional items for: $5 each

FEATURED SELECTIONS

		Total COST of $9.95 items	
Vinegar Formula Guide	This one-of-a-kind, ground breaking book gives you exact formulas and measurements for ALL of your vinegar applications! In it you'll find step-by-step, easy-to-use instructions for home health remedies, cleaning projects and more!	$19.95	
Hydrogen Peroxide Formula Guide	FINALLY...No more guesswork! Step-by-step instructions and specific measurements for hundreds of amazing hydrogen peroxide uses. Learn how to use hydrogen peroxide to clean your home, balance pH soil levels, use as a home remedy or beautify your life! It is all here!	$19.95	
The Cinnamon Book	Research studies have found this amazing spice is loaded with health benefits. Find out how cinnamon can be used in treating common (and not so common) conditions such as diabetes, obesity, arthritis, high cholesterol and a host of other ailments.	$19.95	

Order any 2 or more Featured Selections for only $10 each...	Postage & Handling	$3.98*
	TOTAL	

* Shipping of 10 or more books = $6.96

90-DAY MONEY-BACK GUARANTEE

Please rush me the items marked above. I understand that I must be completely satisfied or I can return any item within 90 days for a full and prompt refund of my purchase price.

I am enclosing $_____ by: ❏ Check ❏ Money Order (Make checks payable to James Direct Inc)

Charge my credit card Signature _____

Card No. _____ Exp. Date _____

Name _____ Address _____

City _____ State _____ Zip _____

Telephone Number (_____) _____

❏ Yes! I'd like to know about freebies, specials and new products before they are nationally advertised. My email address is: _____

Mail To: **James Direct Inc.** • PO Box 980, Dept. A1412 • Hartville, Ohio 44632
Customer Service (330) 877-0800 • *http://www.jamesdirect.com*

THE MAGIC OF BAKING SODA

We all know baking soda works like magic around the house. It cleans, deodorizes & works wonders in the kitchen and in the garden. But did you know it's an effective remedy for allergies, bladder infection, heart disorders… *and MORE!*

THE VINEGAR ANNIVERSARY BOOK

Handsome coffee table edition and brand new information on Mother Nature's Secret Weapon – apple cider vinegar!

AMISH GARDENING SECRETS

There's something for everyone in *Amish Gardening Secrets*. This BIG collection contains over 800 gardening hints, suggestions, time savers and tonics that have been passed down over the years in Amish communities and elsewhere.

THE MAGIC OF HYDROGEN PEROXIDE

Hundreds of health cures & home remedy uses for hydrogen peroxide. You'll be amazed to see how a little hydrogen peroxide mixed with a pinch of this or that from your cupboard can do everything from relieving chronic pain to making age spots go away! Easy household cleaning formulas too!

THE VINEGAR HOME GUIDE

Emily Thacker presents her second volume of hundreds of all-new vinegar tips. Use versatile vinegar to add a low-sodium zap of flavor to your cooking, as well as getting your house "white-glove" clean for just pennies. Plus, safe and easy tips on shining and polishing brass, copper & pewter and removing stubborn stains & static cling in your laundry!

VINEGAR FORMULA GUIDE

Studies have shown vinegar to be effective at not only cleaning and disinfecting, but also as a natural home remedy for conditions such as lowering cholesterol, fighting disease, easing arthritis, improving circulation and more! Now learn the exact formulas and measurements for EACH home remedy and cleaning project in a concise, easy-to-read format! No more guesswork!

HYDROGEN PEROXIDE FORMULA GUIDE

This unique book lists hundreds of home remedy, gardening and cleaning uses for peroxide along with exact measurements and instructions for each use. No mistakes and no guesswork!

THE CINNAMON BOOK

Cinnamon is rich in natural healing properties such as being an anti-oxidant, anti-inflammatory, anti-coagulant, anti-microbial, anti-parasitic, anti-tumor – just to name a few! Find out how cinnamon can be used to fight everything from simple cuts and scrapes to chronic health condition, safely and naturally!

* Each Book has its own FREE Bonus!

Index

168